composing myself

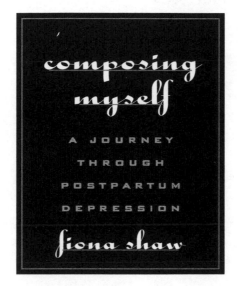

composing
myself

A JOURNEY
THROUGH
POSTPARTUM
DEPRESSION

fiona shaw

STEERFORTH PRESS
SOUTH ROYALTON, VERMONT

First published in England in 1997
by Viking, as *Out of Me: The Story of a Postnatal Breakdown*

Excerpt from "The Cellar of Memory" by Anna Akhmatova, reproduced with permission from *The Complete Poems of Anna Akhmatova,* translated by Judith
Hemschemeyer and published by Canongate Books Ltd., Edinburgh, 1992.

Excerpt from "Sestina" from *The Complete Poems 1927-1979* by Elizabeth Bishop
copyright © 1979, 1983 by Alice Heron Methfessel. Reprinted by permission of
Farrar, Strauss & Giroux, Inc.

Library of Congress Cataloging-in-Publication Data
Shaw, Fiona
[Out of me]
Composing myself : a journey through postpartum depression / Fiona Shaw.
p. cm.
Previously published by London's Viking Press in 1997
under the title: Out of me : the story of a postnatal breakdown.
Includes bibliographical references.
ISBN 1-883642-97-3
1. Shaw, Fiona—Health.   2. Postpartum depression—
Patients—England—Biography.   I. Title
RG852. S5   1998
618. 7'6—dc21
[B]   97-50162
CIP

Manufactured in the United States of America

FIRST AMERICAN EDITION

For Eliza and Jesse

contents

Hold Me Now   1
Planting Tears   93
In Search of an Illness   143
The Desk   189

Bibliography   203
Acknowledgments   209

But it is pure nonsense, that I live grieving
And that reminiscence gnaws at me.
I don't often visit memory
And it always surprises me.

ANNA AKHMATOVA, "THE CELLAR OF MEMORY"

One need not be a Chamber — to be Haunted —
One need not be a House —
The Brain has Corridors — surpassing
Material Place —

EMILY DICKINSON

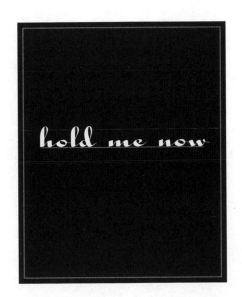

IF YOU OPEN THE DOOR of the house, what do you see? It depends what you look at. To be sure, this is a kitchen you are walking into. It has the paraphernalia of such a place, in its own way. It's quiet right now, its inhabitants have left you to see it as you choose. An odd task, you might say, just to describe the room. How much can be told this way?

Perhaps you are someone who has already stroked the flaking green paint of the splashboard with a surreptitious toe before opening the front door. If you are, then maybe you notice the paintwork as you enter the room, can tell it was done in a rush, and not by professionals. You spot the places where it hasn't fully covered and where the little smears were never quite wiped from the edges of the windowpanes. And look down at the yellow pink of the terracotta tiles, testing their surface with your finger. They are dusty and still porous, never properly sealed. The marks left on them by oil, wine, coffee, milk, and spats of food trace the routes around the kitchen, their odd-shaped spillages like a series of archipelagos.

As you walk the length of the room, you notice the old plaster on the walls with its cracks and bulges and guess that the cost of the new was reckoned with. Your single glance takes in the spaces where the cupboards, not yet made, will go one day, filled now with a child's trolley, a basket of vegetables, the cat's dish. You figure out quickly that this one room used to be two, and not that long ago, from the lay of the joists across the length of the kitchen. There is the old door, now a windowseat. The borrowed light set in the opposite wall is a canny device to brighten the long, low-ceilinged room. And so you go on, estimating, calculating the shape of things that were.

Open the door again and what do you see? This time your eye is caught by the cobwebs clutching the corners of the room and the shiny dry streams made across the floor beside the window, where the snails come out at night to play. Catching your foot on the cat basket pushed close to the Aga stove, you interrupt the meditations of half a dozen silverfish and they shiver their way out of sight, hack into another darkness. There are bread crumbs on the table beside the Aga, still soft when you lick a finger for them. And a heap of books, all sorts, and newspapers. In the sink, one of those old,

white, vast farmhouse affairs, is a pile of dishes, stacked waiting. Breakfast for two people. One of them must be small,
their unbreakable plate just visible beneath the china, and a
plastic bib leaning up against one half-full mug of coffee, its
pelican jowl still pooling spent milk, cereal, and a piece of
toast flecked with red.

It seems that someone must cook in this room, though
nothing is fitted to anything else. There is a pantry, for
heaven's sake, and a high shelf with pots and pans, quite visible. An old-fashioned set of scales and kitchen implements
hangs upon the wall. It's like hanging your underwear out
in public, this display of knives and peelers, whisk and fun-
nel, grater, fish knife, palette knife, and ladle. Why everything
hasn't been neatly fitted, tidied away, you can't imagine. And
the clock on the wall has stopped. It is no longer a minute
before twelve.

You weigh up the washroom, visible through the borrowed light. What kind of woman runs this house? All the
apparatus of the well-ordered life is there, ready to sweep
and scrub, wash and chasten the dirt and dust of the old cottage. Perhaps there's no reason to doubt that this house is a
safe one, if too dusty for your taste and showing off just
those things you like to keep behind closed doors.

Open the door once more and what do you see? Now
you are someone who wanders with a different eye. The walls
of this long room are yellow, a paler yellow than the soft stone
of the outside wall. And the doors are all green. There are
small finger marks low down on the paintwork as though
some tiny person has caught their balance on their way
through the room. Bottles of oil on the windowsill — olive,

sunflower, walnut — a bowl of garlic cloves, vinegars, and mustard. Somewhere there must be lines of spices. Small shelves high on the wall near by are tight with books. A few about birds, wildflowers, and trees, but most are all about food: Italian, Indonesian, French, English, Irish recipes; the history of fish and of bread.

A door on one side of the sink opens to a pantry and its stacked delights. A stretch of marble at one end, cheeses easing on its cool caress. Beneath, a rack of wine and other fillips to the spirits. And before you is an array of spices, dried herbs, pastes and purées, rice, pasta, flours, and flavorings. Things pickled, dried, and preserved every which way. Little respect paid to the orthodoxy of any national palate, here are the rudiments of many feasts. Like Aladdin caught unawares, you catch your breath in this cave of delights. But no genie is at home to hear your wish.

Looking down the length of the room, your eye is caught by the pictures at the far end. There is a woodcut of owl and pussycat, the words of the bong tree dancing round about, and dedicated to Eliza, whoever she might be, and another only inches high that looks from afar to be of the nativity: fine-chiseled silhouettes with three kings in tiny flight. Two larger frames hold satirical prints — plump and bustled figures, unsightly even from a distance. You walk toward them, guessing already at the ancient cartoonist. Pass the dresser stacked with plates and cups all colors and sizes, old and new. A table, newspapers and books piled at one end. A high chair, painted red, stands in one corner. Beside it a push-me-pull-you trike, so close to the ground it's hard to imagine legs small enough to sit astraddle.

Postcards rest in each pane of the borrowed light, two lines of six. They make an eclectic picture gallery. Turn a card and there, an unknown script dances a figure round your absent host. Read each one, the dip and flutter of different inks, and overhear the cadence of twelve different conversations, each one started before and played out beyond the card. Then your attention is caught off balance. A photograph, dated on the back. Man, woman, and small child grouped against the pitch of beach. The sea is one blue, and the sky another, as though backlit by the dropping sun. They stand, looking bold before the elements, hands clasped around bucket, spade, and one another. The young woman's dungarees are taut yellow over the swell of her stomach. "Her time must be near," you think, "this woman with another baby in her belly."

❖   ❖   ❖

Now I will recall a night just over four and a half years earlier. It's February and two people arrive at the same cottage. Hugh looks younger than his years and I look younger again. We laugh as rain pours and thunder shudders, running out and in to unpack a heaped car. The cottage is about to become our home. Exhilaration and apprehension mix on Hugh's face. Walking round the empty rooms my eagerness rises, so keen am I to inhabit this place.

It smells of someone else. The rhinoceros-like woman we bought it from. She lived here for thirty years and though she has taken everything else away, she has left her odor. It inhabits the curtains and carpets and tatty kitchen linoleum. We sleep that first night on a bright pink carpet, the next night on floorboards. We tear the smell out of the house, and the dust of someone else's discarded life rises from the floors and sloughs off the ugly hardboard pelmets as they are ripped carefully from the windows.

The February before, our plan was quite different. We would move to London and live in some distant part of the metropolis, hemmed into some small place by all Hugh's books. Hugh was to find another academic job down there and I, well, I don't know. No more studying. Finish my M.A. and then, perhaps, try for something in publishing, or the media. Hugh drew a little sketch: two cartoon figures, one him and one me, and around them four buildings. Terraced house, London basement flat, Edwardian semi-detached and, least likely of all, a cottage with roses growing. Given the improbability of our love affair, perhaps we should have known we'd get the roses (though we had to plant them ourselves).

Lecturer meets student — that's a cliché. Gay man in his mid-thirties meets twenty-year-old fundamentalist Christian woman — not such an obvious alliance. But we fell in love and, once we got over our surprise, fell into bed. We did that in a time-honored way. Together for an evening in London, I missed the last subway home one night. Hugh was staying in a friend's apartment. So she found me something to wear and set up separate beds that night. When she discovered only one was rumpled, she was outraged. We'd not told her how things lay. And then she prophesied, to our separate astonishment, that one day we'd be married. Nothing could have been further from our minds that morning.

Our shared and different virginity amused us, the source of many jokes. How could we compare notes when I had only God to go by and Hugh such a plethora of mortal men? I had been warned of, but not warned off, him before we ever met. "Don't fall for him, he's charming and funny, but he's gay."

We'd been lovers for a while when Hugh found another name for me. He called me "Finn." The name held me. Since early childhood I'd always wanted a name that didn't declare my sex. It seems something of a paradox that this person, who first discovered and then celebrated my body as a woman's body, should also find a name for me that articulated my sexual equivocation.

Once I had fallen, I discovered I was ruthless in love. No matter that we were years apart, no matter that he was living with a man and they'd been ten years together. I didn't fear, as others do, that he would never leave his other life, nor did I care for a second that gay friends disapproved of his defection. His close friends were not surprised.

And what of my religion? My fall from one kind of grace seemed as natural to me as Hugh's from another. My disaffection had been a long time coming. Hugh offered me a crown for it — more than it was worth. The only sadness was to lose my friends. All went. One love affair died, with God, and another was born, not from its ashes but despite them. And in the pleasure of it I didn't stop to think for long about what kind of strange exchange I'd made.

One day, not long after he drew the cartoon, Hugh read me a poem in bed. He began, "Although it is a cold evening, / down by one of the fishhouses / an old man sits netting." And as he read, I fell in love again. This time, though not fashionable to do these days, it was with a poet. The cadences, the translucent phrasing of Elizabeth Bishop's poetry, seduced me. Something else there was, too, something pushed far back behind the eyes. That I would see only years later, when my life had spun me about as I never could have imagined that morning alone in bed with Hugh.

So we never moved to London, but lived a while longer in borrowed spaces. Hugh taught students in the same university as before and I returned to write about my poet. And soon we chose the cottage, roses, thorns, and all, in which to shape a life.

This cottage was divided in two. Two different houses, two front doors, separated by a wall a meter thick. One half we lived in and the other stayed empty. That empty half still had a rusting copper, smelly toilet, and dirty mustard-colored range not old enough for charm. The walls were pasted with paper stuck vertiginously, at odd angles to floor and ceiling. Old designs, floral, animal, even brick, one fusty layer upon another. Scratch the surface with a fingernail, and beneath the sloughing zigzags you might find an ancient puppy, or violets under bricks that never should have eluded decay till now. It was disconcerting to gaze at the walls too long. Ceilings of old limewash showered an ancient charm on this side. Beneath them, the empty rooms became a repository, a place to hold books and junk and dark.

Friends visited and were, between themselves, a little daunted. Of course, our enthusiasm lent enchantment. But if it was a dream cottage, then the dreams were firmly in the heads of its two inhabitants. The place might have been pic-

turesque, but it was also tatty and full of veneer, the cheap fabric of deception, the modernity of the sixties already looking
prehistoric. Windows and wiring needed replacing, it was
cold and drafty with no carpets. And there was so much hardboard, plywood, polystyrene, and wallpaper. Though they
could be ripped off, such appearances, as I discovered, can be
structural. I bought two pairs of overalls and between us we
set about routing the past. Gradually we inhabited this place,
with its multitude of rooms. I was often taken aback that I was
not living my life in the city where I grew up, but in a long,
low cottage in a small country village. I spent many of my
days in my study or in overalls and I loved it. I like anomaly,
and there was no shortage of it.

The cottage had a garden, drystone-walled and full of
shrubs, conifers, and concrete. After a morning in my study
with my fingers on the keys and my head in books, I plea-
sured myself with a sledgehammer and pickax. I wielded
them to a chorus of horror from old men who'd lived there
all their lives, delighting, as ever, in testing my physical
strength to the limit. Some of these onlookers, sucking de-
crepit teeth in disapproval, must have welcomed the advent
of concrete to the village before I was ever born. I destroyed
grey paths and patios and razed a garage in the middle of the
garden to the ground. Where I reveled in demolition, Hugh
became a gardener, as surreptitious in his trips to buy plants
as he ever had been buying books or records. Slowly, over
the years, there grew a wild place of tangled colors, a garden
at once open and secluded, of furtive delights.

Friends came and went, families visited, we ate well, and
there was plenty of wine. We cooked with brio. I'd learned

much from my mother and now, in my own home, I invented my own, delicious meals. My mother cooks for hundreds — every kind of party, wedding, or wake — but eats like a wren. She is small and thin, allowing herself only just what she needs. Self-sufficient, she resents the dictates of her own appetite. I like my own, but suffer my mother's inheritance. So I would perform my own secret masque of self-contempt, cooking up a treat in the kitchen but a storm in my stomach, as you will discover.

All in all, an admirable act of composition. Our life had something of a fairy-tale improbability. Not necessarily to others, but certainly to ourselves. We couldn't always believe our luck. Of course, there was much we'd like and didn't have. But we liked each other and the life we were inventing.

❖   ❖   ❖

So far I have kept a distance, talking about myself almost as though I were not here. I've been skittering across the surface of my life with Hugh, practicing fancy footwork. Now I must stop picking threads and make myself inhabit that elusive first person, tucked away so vigorously, so neatly, somewhere behind a young woman schooled to competence, living obscurely in an English idyll. So please, approach the cottage once more. It is March now, fresh and cold. This time you are walking beside me and I have another tiny figure in my arms.

For nine months I lived with a child in my stomach. I watched incredulously as a small, hard lump rose through

the autumn from deep within my pelvis to spread itself behind my hips and up, till it reached behind my rib cage and
clutched my heart. The first day we discovered this fact of
life, I sat in our garden in the July sun, dazed, as though I
had received a blow, not yet to my body, but to my heart and
mind. I wanted to be pregnant, to have a child with Hugh.
But I found it hard to believe that now an ineluctable journey was taking place. All being well, one day in the spring
someone would be born who would only ever have known
me as their mother. In some sense, my life, too, would begin
again then. Beyond any other identity, motherhood would
become my quotidian.

Between the two of us, we named our comma the sandpiper, nestled deep in my womb, a bird whose delicate, jerky
beak is always "looking for something," in Elizabeth Bishop's
phrase. The bird's feral, twitchy absorption in that shifting
territory where sand and water meet haunted both of us.
And as soon as I could feel its movements in my stomach,
our sandpiper matched its namesake in its endless shifts and
tremors.

I loved being pregnant. My hair was thicker and shinier,
my energy boundless. My appetite, too, was unbounded, except when faced with cauliflower, green salad, pine kernels,
chicken livers, coffee, whisky (an old love), or raisins. Any of
these made me want to throw up. Wearing yellow or black
dungarees and desert boots for most of my pregnancy, I
marched round my life as though daring anything or anybody to break my stride. There was nothing I couldn't do. I
sat at my desk, working on a thesis that would never be
ready before the baby was, resting one hand on my belly

while I flicked pages with the other. This didn't worry me. The thesis had its own momentum and, astonishingly, I didn't doubt for a minute that it would be done, even with a small babe in arms.

It seemed prudent to trade in the pickax for something else. So I exchanged it for a voluminous green bathing suit. Typically, I was as ambitious now as ever, working several times a week to hone my breaststroke technique. By the time I stopped, at about eight months, I could cover the lengths faster than when I had begun. I used to swim at lunchtime, usually in the company of a handful of septuagenarians. Every now and then, some lads would get in the pool and make great play of their talent. I loved to finesse them. First lapping them, then rising like a small whale out of the water and exposing my great green girth.

We decided, that summer of our discovery, it was time to make our two cottages into one. The symbolism seems unwieldy, but there it is. The building work began in January, with the baby due in March. There was deep snow on the ground for much of February and into March, the March I have invited you to return to once more. Outside our cottage the snow mixed with rubble to form a gray, sludgy quagmire, inches deep. Balancing my precious burden, I tiptoed across planks to escape. Inside, the building dust was over all. Even the pots of fresh-made marmalade, tribute to my stubborn, pregnant energy, were covered with a fine film before I could lid them. When our hot water stopped, each trip to the swimming pool became a cleansing ritual as I rinsed the dust of the old house from my hair.

The more frantic my life became, the calmer and more invigorated I was. In the turmoil my unborn child jockeyed for position. At home all day, I was supervising the building work and buying light fixtures, floor tiles, and so on. In between times I attended prenatal checkups and acquired the clothes and apparatus of babyhood. I spent long hours painting and scraping, while still working on my thesis, leaving paint on the word processor keys. One key remained forever blue. I felt myself to be a Renaissance woman, my body pregnant not only with our sandpiper, but also with my own potential.

As our kitchen and bedroom became building sites, we lived, cooked, and slept in the sitting room, surrounded by furniture upended into unfamiliar shapes. Our pleasure in cooking was equally upended as we made our meals on two electric rings, crouched on the sitting-room floor. We ate a lot of eggs and tortellini. Some friends, on finding scrambled egg in the bath (where, with kettles of hot water, we did our washing up) took pity on us. And, like children found out making a den where they oughtn't, we followed them meekly to a house full of hot water and devoid of eggs.

The builders worked to a tight schedule, keen to be out before the baby was. They knew better than we did what such an arrival would mean. So the day before our sandpiper was born, clad as usual in my overalls, I squatted in the cold outside the front door, not to drop my baby, but to chip concrete from quarry tiles. For weeks now my stomach had been tightening in anticipation, so I gave no more thought to its movements than to the weather.

Hermione came for supper that evening. Exerting ourselves, we cooked pasta with anchovies and broccoli on the floor, even grating some fresh Parmesan for our guest. Perched dubiously on what she thought was a chair, she surveyed our domestic arrangements with astonishment. It was hard to imagine a newborn baby swaddled in a corner of this room.

Hugh fell fast asleep that night, and I lay beside him, uncomfortable and awake. When at last I roused him, sure now of what was underway, it was apologetically and feeling obscurely responsible that this wasn't timed better. The baby would be a week early, we joked, more its mother's than its father's child in that. There is a photograph of me in the bath that night. With my body foreshortened, my stomach rises like a flat-topped mountain between my breasts and legs. I look calm, seraphic even, though by then my stomach's clutches were beginning to hurt.

I left a note in the kitchen for the builder: "I'm sorry I can't finish the tiles, but I've gone to have the baby. Finn." We drove through the night to the small cottage hospital six miles away. First the fields, then the streets were empty. We saw no one. Then there were the strange hours, suspended between time, in the delivery room. Just Hugh and me. We had brought a catholic assortment of music tapes to play, something for every whim. Even a bizarre lapse in taste had been accounted for, and my ancient Simon and Garfunkel tape rooted out of a box. But I could tolerate nothing, not Beethoven nor Bob Dylan, not Schubert nor Aretha Franklin. Not even the sublime blandness of Paul and Art. As my labor built, every sound and every touch felt like a haze of needle pricks. Strange, that even when the pain in my stomach was mounting, even when it had me racked in that terrible rhythmic grasp, I could shout out at Hugh's soft touch. I was so hot, but it was all Hugh could do to dab a flannel at my brow without raising a fury from me.

Dressed in a short hospital nightie and no pants, I quickly gave up the dignity of my body and all else to the grip that tore through my middle, down into my groin, and up my spine. Hugh's fear, that squeamishness would prevent him being present for the birth of his child, evaporated as fast as my decorum. He became ruthless with encouragement, urging me on, as though, like my body, he knew in his what was needed now. In those hours before delivery, my baby was forgotten to me. Eclipsed in my mind for the first time in all those months, the creature inside me seemed part of that alien thing my body had become, not part of myself.

I was reading *Dombey and Son* during the final weeks of my pregnancy and I took it with me to the hospital. It sat on a side table, open at page 245 throughout. During those seven hours I never managed to turn the page, but I couldn't bring myself to close the book. As morning came, I walked the room folding myself into the pain every few minutes, though there was no position that brought any relief. The bed in the middle of the delivery room looked like an instrument of torture. I wouldn't go near it except to bury my face in the mattress as though to escape. The midwife, Fran, spoke of "good pains," not with any false cheeriness, but because the more it hurt, the better the labor was progressing. Her Birmingham voice was familiar to me from my prenatal classes. She was young, funny, and without condescension and I had been hugely relieved when she had arrived, declaring, in mock horror that we'd got her for the duration.

It was when I thought I could bear the agony no longer, that my body was going to crumple or splinter, that Fran examined me once again, now squatting on the floor. She told me my time of delivery was near. Suddenly my pelvis felt as though it was being driven downward and every muscle wanted to urge its burden out. Kneeling on the floor, I thought I was splitting in two and needed all Fran's reassurances that it wasn't so. As the baby's head crowned, dark, matted hair and smears of blood, Hugh's words of encouragement to me, his lover, his partner, turned to love murmurs toward his child. And then Fran told me to stop. "Stop pushing, wait, hold everything." How could I stop? Only King Canute had ever asked for more. The baby's umbilical cord was tight around its neck and as I held the tide, I don't know how, Fran cut it and clamped it. It took only a moment and it felt forever.

Minutes later our baby was born and gathered into Hugh's arms. His shirt streaked with blood, his tiny daughter anointed with blood and mucus, this man so frightened of his own squeamishness saw none of it. He had eyes only for the little creature, still curled, in his arms.

The pain stopped. Not slowly, but instantly. And for the first time, I felt my knees go weak. Fran helped me into the chair I had been leaning against and I held my baby. Her eyes still tight shut and fists clenched, she nuzzled for my breast. My body felt dispersed, as though for the time being my arms and legs, my back and feet, had given up the ghost.

Before I'd ever given suck, my baby had sucked my body dry and left me nothing but my love.

So Eliza came into the world. I stayed in the hospital for ten days while Hugh and an assortment of friends painted around the clock, changing the building site I had left back into a home for our new baby. When I walked through the front door with Eliza that Sunday in March, it was as though I were coming into a new house. The kitchen was as wet behind the ears with its new paint as Eliza was in her new life. Yet so far this was simply the life I lived, with my baby and a beautiful yellow room.

❖   ❖   ❖

Eliza was voracious from the first and as incontinent in her diapers as she would later become in her speech. Even when tiny and subject absolutely to the dictates of others, she managed to display that endless, eager, twitchy curiosity that means she is rarely still. Feeding from me, her eyes would rest, holding mine, but her hands and feet were in constant dance. I felt at ease in this new self. Motherhood became me.

Somehow my life as a mother and my life as a student finishing her Ph.D. managed to make way for one another. As soon as Eliza went to sleep during the day, I exchanged runny diapers and runny nipples for the more difficult fluency of my writing. Where before it had taken me half a day to begin as I wound my mind up slowly, now my concentration started as I climbed the stairs to my study. While I was in there I left the mantle of motherhood outside the door.

Then, maybe an hour, maybe two hours later, with the first waking snuffles from Eliza, I was back down the stairs before she'd opened her eyes.

I was never short on frustrations during Eliza's first year. But then I never have been. Even so, in February, just before my twenty-eighth birthday, and pregnant again though I didn't know it, I sat for the oral exam on my thesis. I came out a doctor, though it proved one of the most dismaying conversations I have ever had about my work. My examiners told me at the start that I'd got the Ph.D., but then used the rest of the exam to tell me how disappointing it was. The thesis was divided into two halves. They ignored the first half — a biography — and said there wasn't enough theory in the other, the critique of Bishop's poetry. The thesis, titled *One Art,* was partly about the synthesis we, as critics, can invent between these different acts — of living and of writing. So I felt they'd missed, or chosen to ignore, the point.

Still, to be finished was a delight. A cake was made by friends in my honor, with a sandpiper iced on top. So there I was, an academic doctor in more than one sense. For a moment in July I walked the boards, like my famous thespian namesake. Six months pregnant and dressed in purple, I crossed the stage in gown and hat and took my doctorate in hand.

Tentatively, I wrote around a bit that summer, to see if anyone was interested in publishing what I'd done. Some people were willing to look and see, and I still have hundreds of pages of my thesis beneath my desk, never quite sent off before the baby was born.

We spent a month in Ireland, walking each day to the beaches, Cappagh or Ballyguin. Swimming out into the cold Atlantic, my breath was drawn like a cut from my body. I watched the cormorants hug the water beyond me, sometimes only the beat of their wings visible above the waves. And the terns drop like plummets, the sea receiving them each time with a cursory suck and froth. Then I'd turn and face the land. At the back were mountains, their outlines often shaved by cloud, then bog, small fields with tumbled walls, and finally beach. Treading that freezing water stilled the burden in my belly. Hugh and Eliza were far away and tiny by their sandy castles. I felt calm, prepared. As much a part of this easy, natural, unreflective rhetoric as the birds and the bog. There is a photograph of us on our last evening down on our favorite beach. I am wearing yellow dungarees and a shirt borrowed against the sudden September evening chill. I look directly into the camera, nothing to hide.

During those last months of pregnancy, my only apprehension was for the curly-headed, bleach-haired, rotund and willful chatterbox of a toddler Eliza had become. She knew what was in my stomach, as well as you can when you're only a year and a half out of it. But she seemed unconcerned by my changing shape and unwitting of its consequences. Though a precocious gabbler, matching either of her parents, her sophisticated mimicry anticipated an understanding she didn't yet have. Without thinking of my own past, I grieved for her, that soon she would have to share her parents. It was hard to think she could bear it.

Once again, this time in October, Hugh and I drove through the night to the same small cottage hospital. We took

Eliza to friends to finish her sleep. As I kissed her, I thought I was kissing away something forever, something she would never have again. We passed a little owl sitting on a post. Lit up in the car headlights, it was quite unfazed. It seemed to us a good omen. But all that bird's wisdom couldn't have prepared me for what would happen so soon.

This time around I was reading Elizabeth Bowen's *The Little Girls* and not enjoying it. Unlike *Dombey and Son,* if I didn't finish this during my labor, I knew I never would. It was the kind of writing I could just about hold on to even when the pains got bad. Strange that this was not a mark in its favor. I paced around the delivery room, book in hand, slapping it down when a contraction rose, picking it up sweaty-fingered afterward. I finished it in that room, not long before Jesse, our second daughter, appeared.

She came on a Thursday, first thing in the morning and with a short cord, all just like her big sister, though at least this time the cord was not around her neck. And once again I saw Hugh, his delicate gestures, as he cradled his tiny child, minutes old, and whispered sweet nothings to her untutored ear. I bled after Jesse's birth. An hour after she appeared the flow of blood increased. Sanitary towels were no more than tissue paper beneath this deluge; both my nighties were soaked and my bedsheets blossomed red. Finally I mentioned my predicament to a midwife. Could I please borrow another hospital nightie, I was terribly sorry to be such a nuisance. Suddenly midwives surrounded the bed, blue-frocked and solicitous. All proved to be fine, nothing hurt. But when Eliza arrived that afternoon, no longer one and all alone, I was not allowed to bear her weight upon me.

Unwillingly rebuffed by me, prevented for the first time in her life from climbing onto her mother, Eliza gave her sister a fleeting glance and took off down the hospital corridor. Legging it up and down, from the tank of goldfish at one end to the babies in plastic tanks at the other, she was both exhilarated and in flight. I stayed in the hospital a couple more days and gradually Eliza took in the new view. She held Jesse, stroked her forehead, watched as her diaper was changed, and stared at my breasts as I fed her. Jesse took to the breast like a duck to water, just like Eliza. I enjoyed feeding her, even the ache and leak as I waited for her to wake and eat, my bosom a couple of tight-strung drums across my chest.

Driving away from the hospital on Sunday afternoon I was thrilled with my baby and eager to be back with my little girl. Hugh had made a small wooden toy cot for Eliza. We gave it to her that first night home, complete with doll tucked up inside. She took the babies, real and plastic, in better part, with more enthusiasm than either Hugh or I had dared to hope. In the days afterward, when I had gone again, taking Jesse with me, the little cot still stood in the sitting room for her to play with, a simulacrum to remind that distressed child and unhappy father.

A friend, Kate, was staying with us the night I returned. She gave me a gift that still hangs in our kitchen. Made of a dark metal, it is a votive incense burner to unfamiliar Far Eastern gods. Decorative horses, lions, and elephants dance attendance. If we had known, that night of my return, what dark spirits lay in wait, maybe we'd have lit the incense in a futile effort to appease, though who knew what.

The first few days after Jesse's birth stand like a bulwark against what was to come. For that short time I felt the unique delight and ordinary exhaustion that were already old familiars to me from Eliza's birth. The flowers that arrived smelled sweet, the cards of congratulation, set out on the dresser, spoke true. But in the space of days all that pleasure became vicarious. It was not mine.

The woman who began that week, returning home triumphant with her second child, was not the person there at the end of it, or so it seemed. Where did I go to, or come from? Was the despair I felt when Jesse was ten days old something I had lived with unwittingly? Or something invented out of the blue in that short hour of my baby's life? By then I no longer wondered where my other self had gone. It had never been. There was and could be no other life than the bleak shadowland I now inhabited. Like the boy Augustus in *Struwwelpeter* who wouldn't eat his soup, I was well enough on Monday and by the following Sunday I had relinquished everything. My mind's eye contracted, till it contained only a loathesome vision of my own self.

On Monday I was just a little out of sorts, stuck in a mood of unease that I couldn't shake off. Then I started to cry, more and more often, but I didn't know why. I cried in front of a neighbor, someone with whom I'd only ever been banally cheerful. If Hugh asked me how I was, I wept and had no words. There was no question of parading my new baby in the village, as mothers are wont to do. I wanted to see no one. My mother reassured me on the phone that this was normal after childbirth, maybe thinking of the weepiness people call the "baby blues." I couldn't make her understand, perhaps because I didn't dare describe it to myself like that. It had gone beyond the normal, whatever that is.

On Wednesday Hugh dressed Eliza for a short walk, while I bathed Jesse in the bathroom upstairs. As I heard the front door open, I screamed and screamed, my heart racing with terror at being left alone. Hugh came running, knowing something catastrophic had happened. He had never heard a cry like it. It was the sound of terrible injury and yet I didn't for the life of me know how or where I was injured. He never took the walk but from then on remained within earshot.

I wasn't depressed, I told myself. I had nothing to be depressed about. I simply despised myself. I was making a fuss about nothing, I was putting it on. Why couldn't I snap out of it, pull myself together, in that terrible English phrase? I grappled with words, reaching time and again for any understanding. But though I knew so many, I couldn't find any that told me what I was feeling. The midwives, who visited each day, became worried. Hugh was *very* worried. I retreated further, my face blank with despair. My body became inert, heavy and burdensome. Every gesture was hard. I no longer played with Eliza. It was harder and harder to face her infantile exuberance when I could find no mirror for it. I berated myself, stretched myself on the rack of guilt. How could I deprive my own child this way, why was I refusing to give her the smile she needed?

On Friday I asked Hugh to call the GP. I couldn't leave the house and he visited me at home. A mild case of postpartum depression, he said. There were two courses of action. Either he could put me on antidepressants, but I might well have to stop breast-feeding Jesse (my GP once told me he didn't like breast-feeding). Or I would have to "grin and bear it." Eventually I would feel better. It was not a helpful visit. Breast-feeding my baby was the only thing remaining to me. To stop that would take my last piece of succor. But I could not grin and I could not bear it.

On Saturday I capitulated. The sheets and pillows, bars and baubles of our brass bed became my prison. I could not leave it. My existence was pared away almost to nothing, except for the self-contempt that bruised my eye sockets and throat, that turned my stomach and made my tongue into some large, coarse creature in my mouth. I sat to feed Jesse, but otherwise lay curled, motionless, in some futile effort to still the pain. I longed for someone to take over, for someone, somehow, to mother me. My mind writhed and shifted. It would not be quiet though it found nothing to ease me. Why did I feel like this and why could I not say how I felt? If I could only pretend all was well, maybe it would be. But I could not, or would not. I talked with Hugh, oh so lucidly, I tried to discover why I had stopped my life. And for the first time I could remember, it chilled my marrow to find that words made no difference.

Hugh played with Eliza downstairs. Their noises came up to me like shards of something I once knew about. But I was far from there now. My love for them mixed with hatred of myself, forming a coarse sand beneath the skin. And I twisted on the bed I had made, unable to ease my chafing sores.

Sleep deserted me. And, no longer able to stomach myself, I stopped eating. There was no revulsion but I didn't want to eat anything. Hugh brought food up to me, and took it away again. I would drink only milk in the hope that by doing this I could continue to breast-feed Jesse. I couldn't nourish myself. I was dissociated, watching myself refuse my own life and unable to do anything about it. I capitulated as utterly as I knew how, making myself into some terrible parody of the baby I had given birth to just nine days earlier. Like her unable to leave my bed, like her drinking only milk.

Later that night, Hugh asleep beside me, I wrote down what I could. Perhaps because it gave me no relief, I didn't risk this again in the months that followed. I hadn't kept a diary for years, but found myself somehow compelled to write, to bear witness to my own withdrawal. This is what I set down.

> *24th October 1992. (11 P.M.): Jesse is nearly 10 days old and I am passionately in love with her. My feelings about myself:*
>
> *self-dismay — longing to be mothered — strong fear I'm making all this up — that I've lost my reason for action — wish someone would come in & take all decisions, force my hand — wish to be out of it all, back in hospital even. But horror of being separated from Eliza — fear I'm losing touch with Eliza — fear Hugh won't be able to stand it — incomprehension — desperation — desire for a close friend — fear I'll be unable to give up this condition — boredom & weariness at having to think about it endlessly, never able to*

create another perspective. Everything is sucked into this depression's somber glow — time passing so slowly — not understanding myself — trying to write my mind clear, but it's not going to make any difference — fear of the outside world.

I don't want to see anyone except Hugh, Eliza, Jesse, & the midwives . . .

Everything anybody says feels like another putdown —

What do I want? — the fact that this may all be an hormonal imbalance is no consolation to me — it makes no difference — nor does it make any difference other people saying they suffered post-partum depression or that it goes quickly — so many tears — periods of weeping, about any thing — and then stretches of dried-out numbness — desire to be self-providing, but why — no appetite — no sleep in the day — trying to trace in memory my "back" phase & whether my state of mind was at all similar — Dr. C. said either endure it or take antidepressants, which might mean giving up breastfeeding. I'm not doing that. I can't make myself eat, which is worrying because of Jesse.

I didn't sleep that night. Early the following morning I tried, once more, to explain myself.

25th October (6:45 A.M.): am I just making all this up, to punish myself perhaps? And if I am, why? I can't stand to think of my 2 little girls —

why would I do this to them? Not eating because
I want to clean myself out somehow, yet it's going
to make it hard to feed Jesse. So why do I still do
it, find it so hard to swallow a mouthful?

    Depression is like an amoeba, altering its
shape to take in every corner of my life; just when
you think it's left one place, it turns up in another.
— What is it that makes me, compels me, not to
eat when I know I must, for Jesse? — how can I
talk about it all so volubly with my beloved Hugh
and still be unable to eat or sleep? — it tears me
apart, that I'm going to be unable to feed my Jesse
if I continue like this, but I can't stop it.

It was Sunday now, a week since I had come home. The
life I'd been so keen to return to, to bring our new baby
back to, had gone. Gone was my self-esteem, and composure
had fled. I lay shipwrecked, exhausted, on a rock of revulsion, unable to escape myself. I wanted to abdicate responsibility. I yearned for someone else to take over, to tend me
as I tended my tiny child.

Neither Hugh nor I knew what to do. At our wits' end,
we decided he should call the doctor once again. Though
our GP had offered me nothing, there was nowhere else to
turn. A different GP came out this time. He was gentle. He
didn't tell me what to think nor what to do. He talked with
me for some time, listening carefully as I blurted out my
shame. He didn't tell me to bear it, nor did he try to talk me
out of myself. Then he left the bedroom.

> *Fiona began being weepy on Monday after dis-*
> *charge [from the maternity ward] and has gradu-*
> *ally deteriorated over the last few days. She last ate*
> *2 slices of bread at noon yesterday and is still*
> *drinking. She seems to be caring for her baby very*
> *well and continues to breast-feed.*
>
> *She is a very articulate, intelligent lady and is*
> *well aware that there is a problem. She had previ-*
> *ous eating and depressive problems in the past.*
> *Depression and weight loss while in hospital with*
> *an orthopedic back problem as a teenager and then*
> *[eating problems] as a student. She felt these prob-*
> *lems were cured after her first pregnancy.*
>
> *She cried the whole time I was with her and*
> *blames herself for all the problems!*

This doctor left the bedroom, made several phone calls, and spoke to Hugh. When he returned, he told me he thought I should go back into the hospital. He'd given Hugh a letter for the duty doctor there. At first I didn't understand and assumed that he meant a maternity ward. Then I heard him properly. He was talking about the Mother and Baby Unit of a psychiatric hospital. I didn't associate my state of mind with a psychiatric condition. Then again, I didn't know what a psychiatric condition was. It was a horrible shock to discover I was headed for that dour palace I'd so often passed by on the edge of the city. Later I discovered this GP thought my mood suicidal and that I was a risk to myself. I didn't think of myself as so, though refusing food must be a considerable act of aggression, against oneself as well as against others.

Ten days earlier, I had gathered toothbrush, nightclothes, baby things, and books, my stomach taut with anticipation. Now my stomach was slack, empty, and I had a very different bag to pack. Once again I lifted the red suitcase onto the bed. Once again I filled it, carefully, through tears this time, instead of contractions. Both Hugh and I wandered the house, like characters in a play who don't know their exits or entrances, or whether they are meant to be addressing one another or some other person offstage. Only Eliza kept us in check, needing food, play, and reassurance.

It was cold that Sunday in late October and rain fell steadily out of a bright gray sky. It took perhaps twenty-five minutes to drive to the hospital on an empty road. No one in their right mind would venture far from home on a day like this. There were no small owls to cheer us. We approached the hospital on a long, straight avenue. Nobody seemed to be there. Hugh left me in the car with the children and went in search of a way in. I looked out at a vast Victorian building with many windows. But far from offering any exchange between what is outside and what is in, the windows looked blank. No people showed at them. Surely nothing good could happen in this place.

Eliza chattered out questions. I tried to hide the tears in my voice as I forced out monosyllabic replies. While she was talking of the rain and the trees, all I could think of was the thing I couldn't tell her. That in a short while, I would stay here and she would go. We would be separated and it was my fault. In that car in that parking lot, no kind of anywhere, I wanted to keen for myself and my child, or run. But all I did was sit. Finally Hugh returned, accompanied by a young woman, the nursing assistant in charge of the Mother and Baby Unit that day. She led us around corners, down the side of the building, and in.

We pushed through a heavy door. It closed behind us with a loud clunk, but it wasn't locked. The foyer had a telephone booth in one corner and a bench at the back. Two hospital signs pointed to wards, left and right. We turned right, into the ward. The corridor was long and the ceiling was high. There were doors off to left and right. A few people watched our progress; none of them looked happy. The floor was carpeted in a thin brown, the walls coated pale green. I think there were small pictures on them, the kind you discard from the mind at a glance. We walked past a small, glassed-in office and into a separate set of rooms. This was the Unit, specially built about ten years earlier.

The nursery was large, airy, and drab, seeming to sap color. Walls were papered in brown with grotesque, doll-like homunculi performing tasks in endlessly repeated patterns. It had two windows — one onto the world outside and one onto the nurses' station. The second, curtained only on the nurses' side, was there not for light but for security. It hadn't occurred to me that I might not be trusted with my child. The room was furnished around the edges: four cots, each with a mobile so high above that no baby could see it, four drawers for clothes, four baby baths, washbasin, four low-slung easy chairs, and two white formica tables between them. The place looked cleared for action, though I hadn't figured myself as one of the participants.

At home our children's bedroom was small and intimate, with bright walls, colorful pictures, mobiles at every turn, and a low, sloping ceiling. I was at sea in this unconvincing, institutional replica. When we learned that Jesse would have to sleep here and not in a room with me, Hugh and I nearly left. But even this separation, the crown on all the others, was more bearable than a return home, and in our shared, different terrors, we remained.

The nurse brought a large plastic box of toys for Eliza to play with. Some of them had that waiting-room aura, with too many pieces missing quite to work. Eliza set to, however, with frantic glee. While she played, we drank cups of tea and talked. There was a biscuit on my saucer that I didn't eat.

A young woman psychiatrist came to admit me. Responsive and intelligent, she spent a long time talking with us, reassuring us. Taking notes, listening to everything I said about my past and present, she said she understood the weight of our fear. Of course I was free to leave, of course everyone felt this way about the place when they first came in. Of course the décor was depressing. Insofar as anything persuaded me to stay, she did.

We went to see where I would sleep. It was a gloomy room hard by the nurses' station and out of earshot of the nursery. Though they assured me I would be woken when Jesse cried at night, it seemed a wanton act of cruelty to force me to a bed so far away. On the left of the door, at head height, the wallpaper had been torn and was hanging in strips. It wasn't nice paper, but it looked considerably worse when attention was drawn to it in this way. I didn't want to know what had happened to it, as though it were a sign from a future place too frightening to imagine. There was a surveillance window near the door, again curtained from the outside, two beds, and the necessary rudiments of furniture. I couldn't stay in this grim place. Surely I wasn't the kind of person they had in mind?

Eventually we decided I might as well sleep there one night. It was only the shadow of a decision. There was no-where else for me to go. When Hugh walked out of the nursery with Eliza in his arms, I thought my chest would burst. In my mind I watched her walk that long, pale green corridor away from me, smaller and smaller, until she was just a tiny figure far away and then, gone. I hated myself, that my self-contempt should touch my child.

That evening, alone in the Unit with the nurse, I talked for hours. She brought me a plate of food at some point and took it away untouched. I talked about my family, my father, my writing ambitions. Tears ran from my eyes, making my shirt collar damp. I spoke the same questions over and over, too exhausted by now to find different ways of asking them. Why did I feel like this? Why couldn't I stop crying? Why was I here? Why did I feel so alone? Why had my dad died on me? Why hadn't he wanted me close? Why did nothing make any difference? Why did I simply want to give up? In between the questions, I spoke lucidly, at least to myself. But as before, this multitude of words made no difference.

Walking around the different rooms in the Unit — bed-rooms, bathroom, sitting room, laundry room, nursery — all empty that first night, I felt an interloper. This place must have been built for a different kind of pain. After all, when they asked me where it hurt, I couldn't say. And my bruises didn't show, or so I thought. I couldn't be ill. Not really. In the week that followed I dreaded being found out, discovered beneath my charlatan guise and sent home. How could my misery be legitimate, when it made no sense to me?

❖   ❖   ❖

I don't know how many days and hours I have spent in talking about what happened to me after Jesse's birth and why, nor how many months writing this book. Both the talking and the writing have been vital to my recovery. They have got me everywhere. Somebody told me that not remembering much of this time would be a blessing. They were wrong. I don't remember very much, partly because of my depression, but even more because of the treatment I was about to receive. A lot of the first year after Jesse's birth is blank in my mind. There is nothing more I can recover and it has been like a curse. Sometimes my account will seem disjointed, partial, as I scratch around the thin dust of memories to evoke that time and the months to come. By writing down what I remember, I want to bewitch the curse and conjure a real story out of the sharded, blanked-out nightmare. Not a telltale story waiting to be written, but a tale uncovered from the midst of my awful, collapsed confusion and my leaden return to the ordinary.

In piecing together a narrative, on paper and in conversation, of the broken-down days and months ahead, I have come up again and again against the limits of my own memory — and the differing sharpness of other people's. Having composed what was on my mind, with all its gaps and empty spaces, I have occasionally interspersed my narrative with other people's voices. These include some of my medical notes, mainly written by the nurses whose job it was to watch and care for me, and recollections written down by friends. I was locked into a solitary place and other people's words jar against the isolation inflicted by my mind and memory. They are reminders of how far I had gone in my head, even from those close around me.

What I do remember, I remember sharply. But there are none of those murky shadows of memory, those familiars from childhood, waiting to be grasped and pulled into the light. So, the day after I arrived, I know the day beyond the window was bright. My sister Lucy visited with Hugh and Eliza. Lucy took Eliza outside and they ran with the wind, kicking and turning the leaves, making heaps and troughs in the autumn colors. I stood inside the window, separated by more than glass. Their play was like some language I'd once known but long forgotten. Then they were airplanes, arms outstretched, roaring around the hospital grass. "Why don't we go out and join them?" Hugh's question took me by surprise. It hadn't occurred to me to do so. No airplane could reach the country I was in. But we went out and I put out my arms, a poor shadow of my child, play-acting, not playing.

Hugh brought Eliza to visit me every day and every day I dreaded her departure. Making a virtue of necessity, she quickly invented her own rituals, always returning to the same toys and the same little stash of books kept beneath Jesse's cot. Like her parents, she found it all hard to bear. She threw many tantrums. Often the visits ended when she became too hard to handle and maybe in this way she retained the smallest vestige of autonomy. Though she couldn't decide when to come, and she couldn't take her mother away with her, she could decide when to go. When she'd gone I sat, my legs drawn up to my chest, my throat and eyes throbbing, my body shaking as I wept my love for my daughter.

In those first days I tended to Jesse. I fed, cuddled, changed, and bathed her. I sat in the Unit sitting room, unable to read or watch television, or I hunched on my bed. Hugh and Eliza visited every day, Hugh sometimes twice. He came to see not only me but his tiny, precious daughter. Hiding his grief from me (not hard at the time), he'd cradle his child, who'd been no sooner home, no sooner with him, than spirited away, not by elves or witches, but by her own mother, sucked into the eye of an invisible storm. How much he missed her I never saw at the time, my sight was so turned inward.

Occasionally I took a walk. And in between times I carried on talking, any way I could. My furies were always with me, taunting me ceaselessly: "You're not worth feeding. You must starve." "But if I starve, I'll starve my baby. I can't bear to harm her," I'd reply. "I can't bear to harm my baby. I want above all to feed her." Which meant eating. But I wasn't worth feeding. A horrible circle.

Then, leaving one child, the furies would turn their breath on Eliza. "You're hurting her, she's suffering because of you. You're clever enough, you should get yourself out of this mess. You're not ill, you shouldn't be here." I dreaded being asked to leave and, as these thoughts circled my skull, all I wanted was to curl up in a corner and never come out again. I wanted my dad, dead for eight years, absent for longer. I wanted to be mothered. Some days my chest and head were convulsed by sobs and I went about the ward with my head bowed, embarrassed by my red eyes. Other days my eyes were dry and that was worse. As though I had a huge boil inside me but nothing to lance it with. What would happen if it burst?

I walked from one room to another, one part of the day to the next, wishing I could shrug myself out of my skin and cease, well before midnight. When people suggested to me that I had no good reason for being so full of self-disgust, their words made no sense. I was torpid, a sham, and deserved no self-respect. Most of all I was terribly alone, lost, in a harsh and faraway place, a horrible terrain reserved for me alone. There was nowhere to go, nothing to see, no panorama. Though this landscape surrounded me, vast and amorphous, I couldn't escape the awful confines of my leaden body and downcast eye. I didn't want to live, but I couldn't bear to die. Like the last reach of my terror, the names of my children sounded through my skull. Again and again I would say, beneath my breath, "Oh Eliza, Eliza, my darling, my love, I can't do this to you. Jesse, my baby, my tiny, gorgeous innocent, Jesse."

The nurses seemed patient, willing to listen. I thought that perhaps with their help I could get some purchase on the shiny walls that glassed me into this waking nightmare. Perhaps I could hammer in crampons, sheath myself in a rope of story that would hold good and, clinging for dear life, haul myself from this horrid echo chamber, filled only with the reverberations of my own thoughts. Who knows whether anybody else could have given me the wherewithal to make my bid for escape. But anyway, I soon realized that the nurses were not going to help me climb. It dawned on me that they were only symptom-spotting. They weren't so much listening to me as listening for signs of danger beneath my words. Anything that might indicate I was a threat — to myself, my baby, or anyone else. "Don't spend so much of your energy in talking," one of them said after about a week. "It won't get you anywhere."

Dr. A., my psychiatrist, arrived unannounced a day or so after my arrival. She sat down opposite me and started asking questions. I liked her but was daunted by her. She was intelligent, with her own kind of wit, but never before had I met another woman on such unequal terms: severely depressed patient meets consultant psychiatrist. It was not an equal contest. Her self-confidence was palpable from the first, while my self-esteem had by now entirely gone.

My first two encounters with Dr. A. took the shape in my mind of classic interrogation, with her playing both interrogators' roles. After the initial sympathetic touch she took a stronger line. When she first saw me, Jesse at my breast, she reined in her ferocity. I wasn't eating, she understood. Of course I must eat and in the meantime I must drink high-protein drinks that the nurses would prepare for me. Anti-depressants were a good idea and I should begin taking them. They worked well for women suffering postpartum depression, though unfortunately they took up to three weeks to take effect. She thoroughly endorsed breast-feeding and the medication was quite safe to take while doing so. In fact, watching me made her feel a little broody. Had I any delusions? Unusual thoughts about Jesse or anybody else? I must understand it would take a little time for her to assess how severe my depression was.

So how long do mothers usually stay in the hospital? I asked. Oh, two months would be an average stay — few are in for less time and many for more, came the reply. I listened aghast. It seemed impossible I would need to stay so long. The thought of being in this building that long was like a blow to my head. And why do you think postpartum depression happens? I asked next. Well, as to the causes of postpartum depression, nobody knows for sure, Dr. A. answered, as though she were talking about the weather and not my life, and continued, it's probably a combination of factors: a traumatic event (the birth) triggering a reaction to past history, perhaps compounded by drastic hormonal shifts surrounding pregnancy and birth. And yes, do talk about yourself, it's a good idea.

It soon became clear, however, that Dr. A. didn't intend me to talk to *her*. Her reputation was based principally upon her skill as a prescriber of medication.

Soon after that we met again. I still hadn't eaten any solid food. Apparently I had joked that if I were to be enticed back to eating, the hospital food was not easily going to do the trick. Dr. A. told me that if I didn't start eating I would have to be sectioned and given ECT (electroconvulsive therapy). Then I would start. It's not hard to imagine my fear. I didn't know what sectioned meant, though I'd find out soon enough: compulsory detainment in a hospital, against your will if necessary. And my only knowledge of ECT was in the haziest horror-story form.

Saw Dr. A. yesterday — now feels reassured by being told she must eat. Dr. A. mentioned ECT if Fiona doesn't start eating.

*Had Chlorpromazine 50 mg X 2 yesterday
— feeling slightly dizzy but willing to take 50 mg
Chlorpromazine at night.*

She asked if I had ever had an eating disorder. I said I had, that I was bulimic for several years, though not recently. But Dr. A. seemed to dismiss this, perhaps because I had never confessed it to a doctor. Bulimia nourishes itself on secrecy and few bulimics seek medical help, but I wasn't in a state of mind to mention this.

Then she turned her attention to my fear of the hospital itself. Now her questions felt like threats. I was frightened of the other crazies and didn't want to go near them. I didn't want to eat with them in the ward dining room. I didn't understand the way they looked and their unhappiness terrified me. I walked down the long L-shaped corridor of the main ward, to the kitchen or the telephone, trying not to notice anybody else's gestures, trying to pretend I wasn't there, or they weren't. My world was awry. I couldn't bear to see other people walking on needles, like me.

Dr. A. never gave me false scenarios, but was always alert to the possibility of there being one in my account. She appeared impatient with my anxiety. Like many people long used to working in such hospitals, she seemed to have forgotten her own feelings when she first came to work in such a place. But for the moment, she conceded, I could continue to bring my meals back to the sitting room in the Unit. A record was to be kept of what I ate and I was to be weighed regularly. Bulimics, anorexics, and babies, like the starving and the glutted, know the logic of feeding in its most violent forms. I was caught up in a strange negative food chain, working to starve myself and feed my baby.

The "threat" worked and I began to eat, minimally. My throat didn't seize up and I didn't hide in the bathroom to vomit. Half a sandwich, a bowl of cereal, an apple, a few mouthfuls of institutional curry if I was being watched, none if I wasn't, and so on. And I still drank pints of milk daily as though somehow my body would translate what the cow gave me into what I gave Jesse. How foolish I'd been, if eating again was really this easy.

Only a few days after my arrival, I was joined by two other mothers, faces mundane and unhappy, not saying much about the phantasmagoria inside the skull. Strange, that I was one of them. Their babies seemed veterans at three months compared to Jesse, still fresh from the womb. Cathy wore fluffy slippers through the day and thought her baby girl had secret powers. She didn't speak much, perhaps not liking the sound of her own voice. She performed her life in the Unit as though a psychiatric hospital was a familiar place to raise a baby.

Now I shared my room with Paula, an army wife. She had the bed beneath the flayed wallpaper. If there'd been any jokes to be had, we might have shared them. Instead, we soon shared strategies for excising the pain. The nurses thought we egged each other on. She wanted to see her other two children but at first her husband wouldn't bring them in. In his eyes I, too, was one of the queer ones.

I liked Paula, but for a while I hated her baby. She cried too much. That flat sound, ignored by her mother, tortured me. As I sat feeding Jesse in the chair furthest from Caroline's cot, her monotonous wail ate into my thoughts, made my muscles tight with fury. "Why doesn't anybody stop her?" I'd mutter beneath my breath. "I can't get away from it and I'm going to go mad." She cried as though there were nothing else to be done with her life.

If I compare memories, how scant is my recall of this year after Jesse's birth, when set against all I can remember after Eliza's. It's as though someone had taken a black brush to my memory and covered the whole surface with tarry darkness, just by chance missing the few bits of canvas I can still see. Though I spent two months in the hospital, I am reliant on other people's accounts to find out much of what happened. And if I were to try and paint a canvas of the six months following, it would still mainly be blank. The hardest part of this is that I don't remember my baby. I believe, I have to believe, that I was as intensely connected to, as passionately in love with her in her first year as I am now; that, even when there seemed to be nothing else, I had Eliza and I had Jesse. But I can't pin up any pictures in my mind.

I've searched my medical notes for evidence of this thing. For evidence of my love, through it all, for my tiny child. Once, when I talk of wanting to take a bottle of pills, the nurse asks, do you want to take Jesse too? And I reply, "adamantly," "No, she's too beautiful to go with me." Otherwise all I'm recorded as doing is feeding or changing or settling Jesse well, or less well. I can construct my closeness to her then only by way of our relationship later, which is as forged as any that I could imagine.

There is a game Jesse plays with a fury that Eliza never has. It's not the game so much as her tenacity that takes both Hugh and me aback. We have to tell, and enact with her, the story of her birth. A familiar project for small children. But Jesse has us, whichever of us, do it not once or twice, but again and again. Hour upon hour of it, if we can bear it. My pregnancy, the journey through the night to the hospital and the owl, the birth. Each detail of the birth must be repeated: the cord being cut, Hugh cradling her, my embrace, her first bath, being wrapped in blankets, her first feed from my breasts. But the most important part of the story, the part that sends her into a rapture and sends shivers down our spines, is the telling of our pleasure. We must say, again and again, how thrilled we were to have our new baby, how happy we were, how much pleasure she gave us. I can say it, confidently, about the first four days. But still I feel queasy because I know what happened next. Perhaps Jesse knows it too, somewhere, somehow. But it will be a hard thing for all of us when we have to take her game further on.

By day, public life in the main ward was conducted along its L-shaped corridor. Pushing open the main ward door and stepping on to the long main corridor, a glance to right and left showed the kitchen and dining room. From the start, I liked the former and loathed the latter. The cleaners were queens of the kitchen, always cheerful, and friendly to me. On my first morning, as I fumbled with the hot water geyser and rummaged the different tubs looking for tea bags, I heard them talk of the tiny arrival in the nursery. When I said she was mine, they treated me grandly. Altogether like someone with a new baby, not someone with a psychiatric condition. The cleaners were set apart, they had something active to perform. The rest of us were meant to learn acquiescence. Other performances were discouraged. Perhaps that's why I liked the kitchen. Something happened there, even if it was only tea and toast.

The dining room reminded me of school. Formica-topped tables, thick-glassed hexagonal salt and pepper shakers, and stackable chairs. The food arrived on a great trolley, metal tubs and vats. The lids were taken off and patients left to cut and thrust for themselves. I usually arrived after the others and the food I would have selected was often gone. Who's to say how much Jubilee Pie or Latticed Tart is due to each? The food had as little interest as I in its own flavors and I was usually quite happy to eat, or not eat, something in place of what was due.

When eventually I dared go in at mealtimes, I was by turns bored and frightened by my proximity to other patients. One man, in about his middle forties, often came to sit at the same table. He was clever, contemptuous, and described himself as irredeemably schizophrenic. He liked to trump every conversation, which he could do with ease, and seemed undismayed by his own "crazy" behavior. But when he mentioned his son, he shook with fear at the thought that heredity held the last card and that he might have bequeathed him this condition. There were other regular eating companions but I can't put faces, let alone identities, to them.

Beyond kitchen and dining room, there were windows to the outside on one side of the corridor, bedrooms on the other. Then a half-glassed room I came to know as the ward-round room and some toilets. Beyond these, a broad staircase marked the corridor's turn. Upstairs there were more bedrooms, a day room, bathrooms I presume, and a laundry room. My only visits upstairs were made to the ironing board there. The place was always full of worn, gray clothes stacked above the washing machines, draped over the clotheshorses. I ironed my things and, just once, my fingers.

At the corner of the corridor's L were a few sagging easy chairs, almost always occupied. When empty, their dips and hollows roughly shadowed a human form: head, bottom, elbows, legs. Like bloodless stigmata, the collapsed upholstery recorded, in these pressure points, the inert pain of its absent inhabitants. People mainly sat. Not much else was done, not visibly. Next to this corner was the main day room. I rarely went in there. The television was usually on and the air was brown and stale. There were French windows at the far end through which people sometimes tried to escape.

Around the corner was the nurses' office, half-glassed, and a last bedroom, the one I first slept in beside the entrance to the Mother and Baby Unit. On the door to the Unit it was written that no one, other than mothers or nurses, was allowed in without notifying the staff. I had a privacy through there unimaginable on the main ward and made full use of it. Fraternizing with other patients was regarded as a sign of mental improvement, and severely encouraged by Dr. A. But I've never much wanted to be good at fraternizing and the inside of a mental hospital was not the place to begin.

Next to the Unit nursery was a small room labeled the Milk Kitchen. The other mothers made up their babies' bottles of formula milk in here, and soon after I arrived I had to do the same, but with breast milk. I was getting too tired

and needed to sleep without interruption during the night,
I was told. So an enormous milk-expressing machine arrived from the district hospital next door. I was to express
milk during the day and the night nurses could feed it to
Jesse while I slept. I sat for hours each day at this machine,
wheedling milk from my breasts. Move the suction cup
slightly to the left and the spurt might get stronger. Angle it
upward, just a twitch, and you could catch another tiny trib-
utary of the wan liquid that fissured so unwillingly from my
breasts. Where Jesse could draw a river with one suck, I
could achieve only a trickle.

There was a dial to regulate the degree of suction. It ran
from 0 to 10. I never needed it higher than 4, but on one
occasion I jigged it to 8 by mistake. For a moment there
were stars as my right breast nearly disappeared up the tube.
However full the bottle, Jesse drank up every ounce I could
express. She always wanted more, so often I was woken anyway to finish off the feed. I loathed the daily pressure of the
milking-machine and petitioned against it. After a time the
machine was returned home.

My first impression of the ward was not displaced, but
confirmed by my time there. Perhaps it is just as well that
my eye was turned so far inward. I soon ceased to notice the
texture of the place.

I favored the night. Though often dopey with sedation
and sleep, I liked feeding my baby then, no one else around
(except the nurse keeping an eye). The darkness gave re-
prieve. The book at bedtime, written in the margins of the
daily horror story, spoke in a melancholy but quieter voice.
After feeding Jesse, I walked the ward corridor, twilit under

muted bulbs, to the kitchen. Making tea there all alone, I could be calm, less fierce.

> *When I visited Fiona in the hospital, I was struck by the competent, efficient, but completely unemotional way she handled Jesse, picking her up, feeding her and putting her down, as one of our friends said, "like a fork in a drawer."*

Paradoxically, despite my need for solitude, and though surrounded by people in the day, I was lonely. I yearned for Eliza's infant gestures, the hugs and wriggles, and I needed Hugh. But when Hugh put his arms around me, I shrank. Each time his gesture spoke of something we shared, but that I couldn't now return or return to. I was too far away. To hug him would betray our old intimacy. No, the comfort I longed for was that of relative strangers. I wanted women to put their arms around me, to hold me in even the briefest gesture of reassurance. But the nurses never touched me, unless it was to prevent something.

It is the job of all nurses to keep an eye on their patients, but of nurses on an acute psychiatric ward, this is uniquely true. I was always being watched, at first more discreetly, from a distance, and later, oh so closely. The nurses' glances seemed impartial and they rarely offered an opinion. But what did they do with all they saw? They checked what I ate, glimpsed my daily phone calls to Hugh, came to find me if I tried to sit alone, sat in the nursery while I fed Jesse, changed her, bathed her, held her. They wanted to know how I felt toward her and they checked our cuddles. They never touched me until I started touching, more than touching, myself. Then, as I began to strike myself, scorch my skin, blunt my thoughts against the wall, they intervened and stopped me. They didn't understand. I had to distract myself from the revulsion battened onto the inside of my skull.

> *Food eaten: One Weetabix for breakfast & a few mouthfuls of meat and carrots for lunch. A bit of potato for tea. Fiona has lost 4 lbs in 5 days.*
>
> *Fiona found very upset . . . Spoke about dreams: Jesse asleep in her arms & Fiona going to put her in her cot & another form of Jesse already lying there leering up at her who wouldn't go away. Couldn't put Jesse on top of that form, leering & looking at her strangely. Dream ended because the real Jesse woke up. Several dreams about her & Eliza going off on their own on long journeys, e.g. them being on a railway track, just going along, the two of them.*
>
> *Discussed further children. Fiona wants another baby quickly. Advised to wait a couple of years. I am worried about this lady and suggest a close eye be kept over next 24 hours.*

If I wanted to walk outside the hospital, I had to do so in the company of nurses or a friend. I didn't want to go home, nor even to flee the hospital. But after a week of all this watching I needed, more than anything, to be apart from everyone, just for a short while. Though tormented by my thoughts, I longed to be left alone with them.

The first walk I took from that place is the only one I remember well. Accompanied by a nurse, I left the hospital and for a brief time walked the city with the rest of the world. Jesse lay in a hospital pram, wrapped in "Property Of" blankets against the cold autumn wind. Drizzle threatened the air. We walked the long hospital avenue, trees making what din they could with the last of their leaves. The boys playing football on the grass didn't watch us, but then we were a little way away from them. When we reached the road I was given the choice: "Which way do you want to go?" Into the city or into the suburbs, I asked myself. So great was my fear of meeting someone I knew, I chose the suburbs. Even so, everyone we passed could surely see I had come from the mental hospital.

I had thought the walk would soothe Jesse to sleep but she was restless in the pram. Though her eyes were closed she flailed her tiny fists, flinched her cheeks. As for me, I breathed this outside air with relief, though it did nothing to ease the claustrophobia in my skull. We walked beside big roads, heavy with traffic, then eased our way on to smaller vales and drives, houses flounced to left and right by net curtains. At one point we walked beside the river, a stretch I didn't know. That made me uneasy, as though the river and I shared an unspoken alliance, one I didn't want to acknowledge.

Asked to go out for walk; we walked along the river. Fiona told me a dream she'd had last night, which thankfully she'd awoken from. It consisted of two tiny, malicious children plotting to kill their

parents. And she had read a book about the chil-
dren, and knew the plot, but was unable to do
anything to stop them.

During that first week in the hospital, many of my closest friends were far afield. The first friend to see me there,
Sara, had herself been hospitalized years before for anorexia.
Only this shared fact made her visit possible. We stood in the
middle of the nursery floor, a big, blank space, and she put
her arms around my shoulders. While I cried, she held me.
To be held was all that I wanted and more than I could bear.

> *She sat in a chair with her knees held against her*
> *chest. A desperate fetal position — more like a*
> *warding off than a seeking for solace. This woman*
> *had changed utterly in so short a time, that was*
> *what was disconcerting*
> *Jesse was asleep in the cot — scrawny and*
> *pale under a drab blanket — I felt concerned that*
> *Fiona would hurt her. Although she said she'd*
> *never do that. How she could not feel Jesse was*
> *somehow to blame.*

Sara gave me a present for Eliza, a book about colors and
babies. Cheerful pictures of babies dressed in stylish pink,
white, black, red, yellow, playing with immaculate toys in
pink, white, black, red, yellow, surrounded by high chairs
and toys untainted by use. Motherless and happy, they
looked like the babies in a fashion catalogue. Eliza loved the
book. It had to be read each day. But when finally I brought

it home, I put it in the trash. It seemed rank with the perfume of that place. Its pristine outlines reminded me too much of the blear-colored room it and I had lived in.

> *While talking she was crouched in a corner of the nursery, hugging Jesse. States the corner is where she felt safe. Very tearful throughout. She feels she is making all of this up. But realizes this cannot be so.*
>
> *Hostile-looking & uncommunicative this evening. Spent periods crouched on the floor in the kitchen, nursery & lounge.*

Two of the midwives also visited me in that first week, both women I liked greatly. But when they sat down beside me, I was delivered into such a storm of fracture and dismay, they decided their presence made things worse and stopped coming. Though I didn't know why, I wasn't surprised. I didn't warrant their attention. In the face of their affection, I had wept out my estrangement. Their comfort was excruciating. Like the skin sweetness of a bitter apple, it promised something I knew I couldn't have more than a moment's illusory taste of.

About three days after my arrival on the ward, I was approached by a slender woman, designer blonde and dressed in clothes with rare labels. How had she found her way to this place? It must be a category mistake. She sat on the sofa opposite me and explained that she was the occupational therapist. I wondered why she had come to see me. I didn't want any occupation. And in a rare piece of performance art at that time, I showed myself off as someone most self-composed. I was in charge of myself and would be out of this place in a matter of days. There was little point in me starting occupational therapy. Though I forgot so much, the memory of this meeting stayed with me and I blushed whenever I met the woman in the months that followed. Strange, that composure should be so much more embarrassing than agitation. Anyway, I don't imagine my performance convinced her as it did me.

I've always subscribed to a robust theory of misery in my own case, in which a bracing walk, good conversation, delectable novel, or strong drink can put to rout the worst of it. Though it's not something I believe for other people, I take a harsher line on myself. In this I guess I was following the family line. But now the pressure in my head was unrelenting and I could find no ease. Eight years earlier, when my father had died suddenly, I used to wake in the months afterward sick to my stomach with something that for a moment I could not recall. Once I had rubbed the momentary stick of sleep from my eyes, I knew the feeling to be grief and that I didn't wish it to go. This time I didn't understand the core of grief I was carrying. Though it shaped itself to my life like an amoeba, I couldn't grasp it.

Five days in I had a conversation with my friend Adam, come up from London to see me and Hugh in our different emergencies. I sat at the pillow end, Adam at the foot, of my bed. He gave me a proof copy of the book he'd just written, a collection of psychoanalytic essays. The slim volume sat on my bedside table the whole of my stay, unread. It kept a connection for me, it became a talisman for the conversations I really wanted to have, the ones that would have made a difference.

> *I embraced you, as usual, when we met, but your body was limp and your face seemed overcast. You took me into your room, as if you were going to show me something but we were momentarily deflated at meeting in such joyless circumstances. It is terrible to see people you love wanting to be able to enjoy your presence, and being baffled by being unable to. You seemed completely normal and familiar to me, but caved in and slowed down.*
>
> *I wanted your vigor back; it was as though I was seeing the underside of that glow of well-being you usually exuded, your extreme exaggeration and extreme generosity. The gentleness of manner you had been reduced to was almost unbearable.*
>
> *When I left you said "Come again when you can . . . soon," and "soon" seemed like an afterthought, a new idea.*

What Adam and I spoke of, I don't recall. I only know we spoke of my father. I was haunted, during those weeks, by two ghosts, that of my dead father and the specter of myself when I was about Eliza's age. That was when my parents had split up, that was when my dad left me. And here I was, abandoning my own daughter. So maybe that is what I talked about. Anyway, something was consolidated in that conversation, something still alive, just out of reach in my mind. As we ignored the paper hanging from the walls, what I became aware of was the violence in my own wishing, the violence directed toward the fabric of my own body.

On the eve of my first full week in the hospital, I had my own Saturday night jaunt. As the light failed in the sky, I opened one of the doors from the Unit and walked into the grounds. Avoiding the clear expanse of grass, I kept to the shadows. Tucking myself beneath bushes, standing under tall trees, my eyes reached for the darkening shapes their branches made in the gloaming. My distress seemed to inhabit the landscape. I felt at home in these shades. I walked slowly at first, then faster, all unobserved, relieved to be still palpable in this world beyond my own head. Then, after half an hour, I returned. No one had noticed my absence.

The following evening I did the same. It was warm outside. The vast hospital building gave no sign of the teeming, distraught life it harbored inside. I felt very much alone, possessed by my unhappiness but relieved to be away from the impersonal and strangely offhand scrutiny of my hospital existence. I was looking for a crisis, though I didn't know what. As it was, my solitary walk proved enough. It went beyond the bounds of acceptable behavior. It was not the walk itself, I think, but the place I was discovered in that made it too much for them to tolerate.

A railway line runs along one side of the hospital grounds. I was standing beside it when a nurse found me. She came running, breathless, alarmed. "Where have you been, what on earth do you think you're doing?" she asked. "Why are you walking here?" I replied that I wanted to be alone and so I'd taken myself for a walk. She thought, of course, that I was considering suicide and led me indoors, quite as though I'd been a naughty child.

It was a coincidence that she found me near the railway line and not beneath a tree. But I couldn't be bothered to refute her assumptions. I was looking at the world through a piece of gauze. Everything out there seemed indistinct and unimportant. In my despair I was beyond caring what others thought about me, passive in the face of the decisions suddenly made on my behalf.

> *Puerperal Depressive Illness. Actively suicidal. Section 5(2). "A" observation: 1. Allocated nurse to be within touching distance and full view at all times. 2. While using toilet, door must not be locked and allocated nurse to remain immediately outside. 3. If Fiona goes missing, search ward, grounds, inform senior nurse, duty doctor and police. Inform relatives.*

I was sectioned immediately. After that, of course, I could never be alone. Someone was there wherever I walked, close enough to touch me with just a single step. When I went to the toilet, I could push the door to but not shut it and I couldn't sit comfortably with the sounds of my bowels, knowing someone was so near at hand. I'd found seclusion in the bathroom before, but now a nurse sat in there with me. How could I stretch my body out beneath the water with someone so close behind? When I went to bed, the door remained open and just outside I could see a figure seated on a chair, in view of my dreams.

I walked the long corridor each morning to phone Hugh from the pay phone in the foyer (he brought me a daily stock of coins). And at my back, or at my side, walked somebody else. When I spoke on the phone I hunkered down and into the wall as far as I could, turning my back, while my minder stood scant footsteps away. Now every time I passed a door to the outside, I wished myself away. I became furtive, scrabbling for a little privacy, boxed between a horrible interior, where I was sole inhabitant, and a world beyond that wouldn't let me alone.

For a short while I was caught in the trap of good behavior. I couldn't choose my company, never knowing from one nursing shift to the next who I was going to have beside me. Some of the nurses I liked and some I grew to loathe, finding their proximity unbearable, their remarks stupid, and the looks they gave me insidious and disapproving. Nevertheless I felt obliged to be polite to them. After all, it was rude to spend hours in someone's company and not talk. When Hugh came to visit and the nurse on guard backed off a little, I tried to describe how oppressive it was to have to make conversation in this way. Then even this decorum ended. The conversation seemed to be over, though I'd never managed to have it.

I would sit on the swirly sitting-room carpet with my back to the wall and my knees drawn up to my chin. Or else in my bedroom I could pull my bed a little way out from the wall and make a niche just my size on the floor. Wedged between two easy chairs, or between the television and sofa, or the bed and the wall, I was enclosed. If the kitchen was empty and I could go no further, I huddled down in a corner there.

My follower was always close by, but wouldn't stop me at this point. Sometimes I clenched my hands tight across my knees, breaking my grip in the end only to grab the furniture as they pulled me apart.

Now I began to hit my head, against the wall or bed frame, cupboard or chair. At first it was little more than a vibration, invisible almost, reassuring, like a hand stroking my skull. Then it became a gentle rocking motion. "Why are you doing that, Fiona? That isn't the way to help yourself, is it? Please don't." Once they started questioning me, I had to act fast before I was stopped. I shut my eyes and let myself go. Harder and harder I brought my head against the wall's cold cheek until all I could feel was the bruise in my skin. "Stop it, Fiona, stop it now. Stop banging your head or I'll have to prevent you." The nurses tried to hold their tone calm, but only a few could keep my urgent rhythm from their voice.

If I could find that sharp edge of physical pain before I was stopped, then it would distract me for a moment from the other one. My muscles clenched — arms, legs, stomach, and neck tight — as I sought relief. And for a few precious moments I could think of nothing but my head on the wall. Then somebody's hands were on me, tugging at my arms, pulling me away, holding me from it.

> *Has been banging her head and digging fingernails into back of her hands.*
> *Found with large hair grip which she was trying to break in half wanting to gouge at herself. Has scratched herself at every opportunity.*

Talked about her dad: leaving her at same age as Eliza is now; he just went round & round in her mind.

Little short-tempered with Jesse this PM, not wanting to change her dirty diaper, wanting to watch the news instead.

Again and again I returned to the wall. I had eyes only for my own pain. When I was held off, it made me angry. If I became too unmanageable, I was given medication early. Sleep was held out to me like a lollipop to a child and in the end I popped the hated pills.

At first I was given sedatives, then after about a week, antidepressants too. The drugs seemed beside the point, but I took them, unwillingly. They were all quite safe to take while breast-feeding.

Jesse was a wizened dopey little creature who very quickly developed a rash of spots from whatever drugs she was taking in with her mother's milk (though the hospital had assured F that the drugs she was taking would have no effect on the baby).

When after several weeks both Jesse and I came out in a violently itchy rash all over, I was changed to another sedative. No one apologized and, slumped deep within my depressed inertia, I didn't protest.

Persistent truncal rash — change Chlorpromazine to Trifluoperazine.

I made one furtive attempt not to take some pills, putting them behind my tongue instead of swallowing them, then throwing them away when no one was looking. Nobody said anything to me, but the pills were replaced by a vile-tasting liquid. I had no choice but to swallow. It left a horrid taste and a burning sensation in my throat that I couldn't rinse away. I promised not to be naughty again. I pleaded for the pills to be restored and after a few days they were. I was humiliated. Sectioned and deeply depressed, I had no power to refuse my treatment directly. But they should have dealt directly with me, spoken to me like an adult and warned me rather than treating me like a small child. The drugs made me dizzy, dry-mouthed, and slow. Maybe they helped to prevent me from making any serious attempts to hurt myself, I don't know.

My strategies for self-injury were only skin deep. I never actively tried to kill myself. All I sought was that brief rush of the nerves that made me forget for a moment, as my body tried to accommodate some small thorn in the flesh. So I scratched myself with my nails till skin burns tracked along the backs of my hands and up my arms. This pain I could achieve with the smallest movement of my hands, hard for the nurses to see or prevent.

Fiona had stuck a diaper pin through her r. wrist. Told me she did same thing when in hospital aged fifteen; it helped take her mind off other problems.

Soon after Adam's visit, the first burns already scabbing above my thumbs, I asked Hugh to bring me a pair of nail scissors. After giving them to me, he felt uneasy and told the nurses. I had put them in my bedside drawer, a resource stored away in case. When I was asked for them, I handed them over. My argument was not with the nurses but with myself and I acquiesced in most things.

Only once did I manage to iron my clothes unwatched. When I had finished the last shirt, I had my reward. I laid the heated metal down upon my little finger, kept it there for a moment, and then breathed out a gasp. The burn didn't show until the next day. When asked how I came by the angry red blister stretching across two knuckles of the finger, I explained. I wouldn't be able to repeat it, my minders hung too close by then.

In the kitchen was a large urn, always full of boiling water. This offered easy, quick fixes of pain. One course of water over my hand was usually all I could manage, without my attendant moving in, suspicious as to why a cup of coffee took so long to fill. Still, in my scale of negative esteem, the scald was worth it.

Continues headbanging, scratching hands. Admits to putting her hands under the scalding geyser in the kitchen.

"Why don't they give her ECT?" the nurses would say outside my door, close to tears. "It always works for these miserable mums." I didn't hear their plea, though by now I wouldn't have cared if they'd said they were going to

lobotomize me. Hugh bore all the worrying and he remembers their words.

By the time I was put down on the ECT schedule, Hugh,
like the nurses, could see no other place to go to. Though
he'd always been deeply suspicious of ECT and acutely aware
of the arguments against it, now he, too, found himself ac-
quiescing with the hospital.

Nobody explained to me what it might do to my mind.
"It isn't painful and it might disturb your short-term memory a little," I was told. "Nothing more." This was at best
misleading. What was meant by "short-term memory"?
What I knew of that day, or the days just before or after? Or
did it refer to weeks of recollection? Did the "disturbance"
mean I would be confused, or lose my memory? Would I recover the memories that got lost, or would the ECT mean I
didn't care about them? I have plenty of questions to ask
now. I had none then.

Maybe the hospital's recalcitrance was a form of damage
limitation. I suspect so. Nobody knows how much memory
might be lost, but if they told you this you might try to refuse
the treatment. By talking vaguely of "short-term memory
disturbance," a patient can't say they weren't warned. I wasn't
warned, however, of the devastating effect it would have on
my memory. ECT cauterized it.

> *ECT (1) Bilateral 1 × 3 seconds. Modified Grand
> Mal fit: 25 seconds.*
>
> *Angry this morning because she wants to be
> able to conquer her illness herself — said she felt
> she was going to the torture clinic this morning.*

Twice a week, for four weeks, I was taken to a special place and there, my hand held, an electric shock was put through my skull and a grand mal fit induced. "Don't worry," one nurse reassured me, "you won't do anything funny while you're in there." As though I would worry about what *I* did while unconscious, rather than about what was done *to* me. From midnight the night before I had to stop eating and drinking, in preparation for the general anaesthetic the following morning. The food was no problem. But I got very thirsty breastfeeding Jesse. In the small hours of the night, my baby at my breast, I longed for a cup of tea or a glass of water. By nine o'clock the following morning my mouth was doubly dry, parched with thirst as well as with dread anticipation.

Although a muscle relaxant is injected along with the anaesthetic to control the patient's convulsions, they need to be sure that any rogue spasm has plenty of room. So I was instructed to wear "loose clothing." This was no difficulty because all the clothes I wore after Jesse's birth were "loose." I wanted to hide my body away. I had one skirt in the hospital so dense with association that I threw it away some time after I left, and two pairs of Hugh's old corduroy trousers. My shirts and sweaters were large, so they could be hitched up discreetly while breastfeeding. And my self-regard didn't permit jewelry. I only wear jewelry when I like myself.

When the message came, I walked the long ward corridor with both the other mothers, also in "loose clothing," and our three attendant nurses. At some point we joined forces with any others from the main ward also going to be shocked. A genteel lady in her early sixties often went with us. Her endless courtesy enraged me. I felt obliged to reply, in surly kind, to her "Good morning," when actually I wanted to curse her. We made a pathetic group, trundling with dread toward our appointment, surrounded by the chivvying cheerfulness of the nurses.

Out through the heavy ward doors we went, through the foyer with the telephone and, for a moment, out of the hospital. Four steps across tarmac, then through a door opposite into the main hospital building. We walked several long corridors, turned a few corners, until we came to a set of double doors. We had arrived. Like a chamber of horrors, there was one set of doors for entry and another, around the corner, for exit. To make sure that those who were about to receive caught no sight of those just shocked.

Inside, the décor was bland and upholstered. No foam or rubber up the walls, but carpet. We all behaved so well. The waiting room had magazines and easy chairs. It was a cross between a dentist's or doctor's office and an airport lounge. As though they couldn't quite decide whether we were going to take the flight or take the medicine. We sat in the easy chairs, not reading the magazines, and one by one we were called, together with our appointed nurse. I preferred going first, but so did everyone else. The nurses tried to make it fair.

It was peculiar, going into an operating theater where there was nothing but unhappiness to operate upon. Inside, there was a high medical bed with a bright light above. As I was directed to sit on it, I was smiled at reassuringly by the people in attendance: anaesthetist, psychiatrist, and others I think. Then I felt scared. I'm quite tall, about five foot ten, but having to climb on to that bed while they all waited around made me feel small and helpless. I was told to take off my shoes, so they could see my toes wiggle when the fit took hold. My nurse put my shoes in a special basket attached beneath the bed. As I lay there, just to the right in my line of vision I could see a large box with dials on it, the source of all my fear. The headpiece with its electrodes, which left a red mark on each temple for Hugh to see, was never in sight.

While my nurse held one hand, the other was taken by the anaesthetist. With a slight, expert movement, he threaded a needle beneath the skin between my knuckles and my wrist and the last thing I knew was a dense pain spreading from my hand and up my arm.

Consciousness returned in another room. The others from the ward were on either side, muttering and groaning. Once I was back, I got out of there as fast as I could. I'd let them into my head when I wasn't there and I didn't want to stay around this place. More than once I was persuaded to wait on my bed a little longer. The headache was often worse if you tried to get up too soon, I was told.

Sometimes I found my shoes for myself beneath the bed, sometimes I was too dizzy to do so. Then I was ushered by my nurse into another room. With more easy chairs and more carpet, it was like a mirror of the first. Here we all sat again, only this time we'd been through the chamber of horrors. There was a little kitchen appended, from where the nurses brought their charges cups of tea and a large family-assortment tin of cookies.

We all sat around, strangely joined by our separate shocks, but apart in this newest waiting room. None of the

patients made polite conversation and the nurses busied
themselves with tea bags to avoid the stunned silence. Our
complicity in this horrible drama was marked on each of us
— two round red marks on the forehead. I know this because Hugh described them to me later. I didn't notice other
people's heads, nor my own, except for the headache that
sometimes pounded afterward. Locked up inside, I had nothing to say to anybody else, nor they to me.

By now I was itching to get out of here and scarcely had
the patience to choose my cookie. Others seemed relieved by
this parody of a social ritual we were seated in and took their
time choosing between the pink wafer and the vanilla.

As far as I remember, I never talked to the other mothers
in the Unit about the ECT. We didn't exchange stories the
way people do with other traumas, like death, childbirth, or
operations — on the heart, or knee, or varicose veins. ECT
was not a shared experience. Of course it might simply be
that the conversations have gone, because once those electrodes had been placed on my temples, my memory was shot
to pieces. So I don't know whether they, too, lost their way
afterward.

> *Complained of forgetfulness and didn't really know*
> *what she was supposed to be doing . . .*
> *Very confused and forgetful throughout day.*

In the immediate fallout I couldn't even find my way
around the ward. Hugh had to show me the way to the
bathroom one day. Arriving on another, he found me frus-
trated in my bedroom because there was nowhere else I

could go and sit. "What about the sitting room?" he asked.
"We've been in there every day with Eliza in the past few
weeks. That's where the toys are kept." So he led me there
and I stood perplexed in the middle of the swirly carpet.
There was something about the room that seemed distantly
familiar, but I was sure I'd never been in there before.

> *Doesn't like having ECT, finds memory loss a bit
> disconcerting. Still hates herself and doesn't feel
> any different than when she came in.*

Once he saw what drastic sweeps the ECT made, Hugh
started a daily diary for me. It meant that I knew who was
coming in to see me that day and the next, or that there was
an ECT session or a ward round tomorrow. But even more
importantly it told me what had happened the previous day.
So I could at least read that Hermione, or my mother, Kate,
Tim, or Michael had been to see me, though I could find
nothing in my head with which to remember their visit.
Conversations were lost almost before I'd finished them.
Even Hugh and Eliza's daily visits are absent, a litany of
blanks in my mind. I needed them, but I can't remember
them. My days had disappeared, never to return.

> *Hugh had described to me with clarity, pity, and hor-
> ror how she was, what had happened, and had told
> me — for instance — that he'd come in to the hos-
> pital to find her being wrestled to the ground by two
> nurses as she was going berserk and trying to hurt
> herself. Nothing he'd told me, however, prepared*

*me for how she looked. It was as if she had with-
ered. She looked shrunken, smaller, pallid, drained,
at once aged and much younger like a defenseless
child. She looked exhausted and completely terrified:
there was extreme panic at the back of her eyes. And
this was a person who, a few weeks before, when she
was heavily pregnant, I'd been mushrooming with in
the autumn woods. I'd kept looking with admiration
and pleasure at this figure gleaming with robust, en-
ergetic, sensuous vitality. She said immediately, as if
confiding in me something I could not possibly have
otherwise known, "I've just had the worst time of my
whole life."*

I persisted in trying to read during all this. I tried and
failed, repeatedly, to take in Michael Ondaatje's novel, *The
English Patient*. It was a joke, picking up a detective novel
and reading the same page again and again because I never
could remember who had killed whom from one day to the
next. I even tried Adam's essays on psychoanalysis (that trea-
tise on the art of forgetting), but I could hold nothing in my
shaken mind.

Recollection is always shaped by forgetting. It would be
impossible to form memories if, like Luria's mnemonist, we
could not forget. This man, who made his living with his
prodigious memory, was incapacitated by all he could remember. He couldn't get rid of, assimilate, or interpret the
clutter in his mind. But, unlike the mnemonist, with our capacity to forget and to remember we are able to make up a
narrative of our life, to connect the present moment with

the shape of the past. It's a language learned as a child, each of us shaping the syllables of memory to suit.

The loss inflicted on me by ECT went far beyond ordinary forgetting. As though suffering from a form of aphasia, I lost the language of recollection, the capacity to give narrative shape or continuity to my life. I felt robbed of my autonomy, reliant on other people for the material with which to shape any account. So Hugh might come to visit me in the evening and I would ask him whom I'd seen that day and what I'd done. But once he'd told me, I was still none the wiser. Sometimes I'd feel the faintest echo of recognition but that would be all. There was nothing there with which I could shape my thoughts. I had no way of making sense of my condition.

If only ECT brought its subjects out in a virulent rash, or made their hair fall out. Maybe then the doctors would take its effects more seriously. As it is, most people receive the same kind of brush-off as I did. Queries are not regarded as legitimate doubts about the nature and side effects of the treatment, but dismissed as the anxious product of the person's depression. All the more reason to get the electrodes on. When I questioned anybody about the possible longer-term effects of ECT on my memory, I was told it would have none. Yet it left a horrible brand on my mind and memory for another year and a half, maybe more.

❖   ❖   ❖

Two weeks in, the first shock of ECT ringing in my skull, continuity went. What I have left are mostly incidental snapshots of memory, recollections in monochrome, without atmosphere or expression. There is no affect, as a psychiatrist might say. They have none of the contrast of black and white, none of the warmth of color. Were I to make a montage with them, all I'd have would be the static posture of someone who had lost her animation and was living a life by rote. From the start of my breaking down, Hugh was shocked by how much I seemed entirely myself. It seemed more terrible to him than if I had been unlike. But the narrowed, self-hating, minimal self, brittle as a Giacometti sculpture, that he visited every day is lost to my memory once ECT had begun. I no longer remember the shape of my despair. There is only a figure in gray, without thoughts or actions, without a voice even. No rage any more, waxing or waning.

My life in the hospital continued in the same way as before, because friends and medical notes tell me so. But to my mind, I became a cipher of my old self. Almost all I have are occasional voiceless images, so indistinct that I'm not even sure whether they're memories at all, of daily life: sitting on my bed with a friend, bathing Jesse in the hospital nursery, watching Eliza play in the Unit sitting room, eating food in the dining room.

I didn't feel better after ECT. But at some point I did stop trying to hurt myself, more or less. And at another I no longer curled up as much. Now I was allowed out of the hospital with Hugh, or a friend, as bodyguard. I remember the first of these sorties. One Sunday in late November, a month after my arrival, I walked into the city to have a pizza with Hugh, Eliza, and three friends. As we crossed a bridge there was no color anywhere. The water had none, nor the sky. When I looked at my skirt, that had no color either. I was very frightened. The day ends there, in my mind. From what Hugh and the others have said, it's just as well. My exposure to the world outside during that walk proved too much to bear somehow. It's not that I did anything drastic, but before the meal was over it was clear to everyone that I had to return to the hospital as fast as possible. Hugh watched as my body seemed to cave in and my eyes expressed that dead terror he recognized too well now. The ordinary world had proved too much. For a while after this I was dragged back into a realm of imperative self-injury, attack being the only defense I had found, and constant surveillance.

The things I know I remember are easily described: occupational therapy, the weekly ward round, a Christmas trip out for lunch. Although I escaped it for a while, I was advised in no uncertain terms to go to some kind of occupational therapy. My recovery would be assessed partly by my capacity to manage it. Apparently it would mark some return to health if I could spend a morning with strangers I had no interest in, engaged in pointless activities. Never mind that the last thing I wanted to be was sociable, especially on these terms. Nevertheless, in the interests of my own escape, I made the journey down different hospital corridors and was dutifully occupied. Like everyone else, I made a three-legged stool, sticking the legs into the predrilled holes. My only autonomous gesture was to paint it red (varnish was the norm). I gave it to Eliza. It was badly-weighted and constantly tipped her off. Later, we mended it a few times until, thankfully, it broke irretrievably and was thrown away. I avoided the other rote "craft" activities. I can see the same women in the same seats repeatedly making the same objects, but I can't remember what they were. Embroideries perhaps, or basketwork.

The person in charge of the craft room looked like a burly PE instructor. He was a kind man in his fifties, uncoercive and, as far as he was able, encouraging to the people suffered to come to him. With his support I made the beginnings of bookends in the shape of elephants for Eliza and Jesse. After drawing the design with Hugh, I cut them out of plywood with a fretsaw. Then I sanded, undercoated, and glossed them. Finally, at home, we painted on faces and tails. Where the stool was underweighted and precarious, these plywood creatures were loaded. They carried so much hope on their sturdy elephant backs. We knew the funny side to all this, but couldn't afford to catch one another's eye.

I went to a couple of cookery sessions in the "kitchen" along the same hospital corridor, to fill up my occupational therapy tariff. It was December and mince pies were being made. Nearly all the others were middle-aged men and the session was pitched for all of them. I was told how to weigh out flour and how to grease pans. Even in my depression I thought it hilarious that my cooking ability had come to this. I, who had cooked feasts for years with my mother in her catering business, I who cooked delicious food at home with Hugh, here I was, standing meekly and dutifully wrapped in an apron, while someone explained to me how to glaze pastry with a brush. But I submitted graciously to the instructor's advice and took my little batch of mince pies

back up to the ward, feeling like some three-year-old returning from nursery school.

Wednesday mornings always had a particular, tight atmosphere in the Unit because this was the day you knew you'd
meet the doctor, this was the day of the ward round. The
nursing staff seemed as intimidated by the prospect as the patients. We'd sit waiting on our beds as the hour approached,
each of us nervous, though you might wonder, what could be
more alarming than what we were already living with? As
with the ECT, each wanted to be first. The order would be decided upon elsewhere and then for each of us there would be
the summons and the walk, with a nurse, along the main ward
corridor to the room with the wall of frosted glass.

Each time I made the walk I'd feel a blush rise. Though
I was already in a psychiatric hospital, this visit to the doctor signaled still further failure to shape my own life.

Less than a minute later we'd arrive at the glass room.
The nurse would knock while I'd look through at the fuzzy
head shapes that awaited me, as though by seeing them first
I could steal a march on my medical interrogators. At other
times, walking to the kitchen or the pay phone, I'd see heads
through the glass and hear the lowered cadences of voices.
So I knew you couldn't hear the words from the wrong side
of the glass and I knew you couldn't make out the faces
through the frosting. But still, when it was my turn to go in,
I felt uneasy. It was as though the room itself was designed
to remind you that nothing was fully private, nor fully visible in this place.

A number of people raised their eyes with Dr. A. each
time I walked through the door. They were all, of course,

well trained not to raise their eyebrows. There was the occupational therapist, who seemed to wear her elegant
clothes in defiance of this drab, unhappy institution. There
was the ward manager, harried by the role he'd landed. He
seemed to have the unenviable task of keeping all parties —
patients, nursing staff, and psychiatrists — what in the world
outside would be termed "happy." There was the nurse responsible for the Mother and Baby Unit that day and there
was the registrar. He was a gray man, the kind of person
who perhaps came to life only in the presence of a hobby.
There were others too, I think, just beyond my mind's eye.

I felt on trial here: at first I used to assume I'd been found
guilty and I took what I saw as my punishment quietly. I had
Dr. A. acting judge. She always seemed to me less interested
in finding out what I thought or felt than in having confirmed some assessment she had already made. And in that
environment, organized around her own style of communi-
cations, all her statements were self-confirming.

Later I was desperate to prove I was a good and upright
citizen and deserved a reward. Before Jesse was born, we had
decided to spend Christmas in Ireland with Hugh's family
and bought the plane tickets. I had joked with the travel
agent: "How can I give a name for the second child on the
tickets? It's still tucked up inside my stomach." And though,
alongside Jesse, I'd given birth to something so horrible and
unexpected, I'd never let go of my determination to make it
to Cork for Christmas. It became my life's goal and each
ward round the occasion to prove I was capable of achieving
it. After initially pooh-poohing it, then keeping it as a carrot
to encourage me, Dr. A. ultimately agreed to the journey.

By the end of my two months in the hospital, in preparation for my return to the ordinary, I had made several, graded trips home. The first were in the company of a nurse. We drove the half-hour to the cottage in the hospital car and ate soup and homemade bread for lunch, left out for us by Hugh. The kitchen seemed more like a film set than the place where I lived. If I'd tapped the walls too hard, I'd have put my fist through this facade I called home. Next I spent a night at home with Hugh and finally a weekend. Nothing remains of those visits. I pursued these excursions into independence with intransigent determination, as though to look to either side and consider why I'd set my heart on this trip would have been too dangerous. Given what happened after Christmas, I think I was right.

We flew to Cork a few days before Christmas and spent two weeks with Hugh's family. The photographs show Eliza with a stocking on our bed, a Christmas tree and presents being opened, Christmas dinner and a crowd around the dining table. Hugh remembers me as a haunted, unhappy, and elsewhere woman, around whom the family stepped gingerly, as though on needles. About that Christmas, this is all I know — that one sodden day I went shopping with Michelle, my sister-in-law. The rain came down outside and that's all. This goal I'd fought for so fiercely, to be released back into my life for Christmas, has shrunk to nothing and to nowhere in my mind.

On the 5th January I went to meet Fiona, Hugh
and the kids off the 6:20 plane. I'd thought of a
joke, that I would pretend to be one of those official

airport "meeters," so I made a large sign with "The
Haughton/Shaw Family" written on it and stood
holding it up as the people from the Dublin plane
started coming through the doorway. However what
came through the door then was not a person ready
for a joke, or able to notice anything: Fiona came
slowly round the corner looking white, exhausted,
and utterly cut off; with a worn-out Hugh and ba-
bies following behind.

On our way home we were met by Hermione at the airport. As we walked out of the airport, toward her car, I noticed
that a strap on Jesse's car seat had been broken. So Hermione
relinquished the belt on her trousers as a substitute. Although
this was hooked adroitly through and under by Hugh, leaving
Jesse secure, my stomach was caught on a hard barb of anxiety. Jesse was going to be hurt if she traveled in that seat. I finally submitted to Hermione's reassurances because otherwise
we would never have left the airport.

For two and a half months home had formed one half
of my life's geographical dialectic, the hospital the other. I
wasn't going to return to the hospital. But I dreaded coming home. And when it happened, and I *went* home, it was
horrible. My home was no home to me.

I unlocked the green door to our cottage and
Fiona and I trooped in to the cold kitchen.
Giving myself up to my usual relief on surviving
another car journey and arriving home, I un-
packed the heaps of luggage, the travel cot, the

buggy. Eliza whooped with pleasure at finding herself back among her familiar playthings in the reassuring geography of home. It was a moment before I realized that Finn had slumped down on the floor beside the dresser looking drained and shattered. I thought at first she might have crumpled up in tiredness or relief like mine. Then I saw that she was crouched in a state of raw terror, as if horror-struck. She couldn't speak, she couldn't get up, she just collapsed into herself as if struck down by some invisible force that had left her exposed to everything she most feared in the world.

How should I write about the next months? As a series of slashes, or a blank space, perhaps? I can borrow other people's recollections, but I can't find my own. To be sure I remember a few facts, but I have no inkling as to my state of mind. It's like trying to walk around a city you've visited long ago, and finding only wasteland. Where there should be that haunting, distant familiarity, there is nothing. No streets to return to, no pavements or gutters, no hidden facades, glimpsed as you walk by, that recall another time. The population is gone; not even the stringy cats or waiflike dogs inhabit this empty place. I can walk backward and forward across these months and discover nothing. So I am reliant on other people — on Hugh more than anyone else — to remember for me. I have to trust him and others for the significance of my own life during this time. So my narrative becomes sparse now as I kick up the dust in my memory to see what remains.

If I open the door to my house that day of our return, I see nothing. There is nothing to conjure with. Hugh tells me that on our return from Ireland I sank once more into an abjection terrifying for others to see. I was frightened of myself, unable to do more than just keep my head above the suck of despair. Now I was visited by a different psychiatric bandwagon. My home was in a different health trust than the Mother and Baby Unit. Since I was no longer an inpatient there, it had nothing more to do with me. Instead I was visited several times a week by an intelligent, sympathetic psychiatric social worker. He would smile, but not as though he expected me to return it. Once he arrived as I was peeling garlic and he showed me a shortcut for removing its papery skin. I asked him whether I could see a psychotherapist, or psychologist, on the National Health Service. He thought it was a good idea, but advised me to wait a while because I was in too vulnerable a state to take the consequences right then.

My health visitor visited regularly, but I dreaded those times when I felt I had to listen to her family problems. We even had a local authority home-help for a short while. She was willing to do anything and I asked her to do some ironing. But she was too cheery and her visits became an endurance test. She insisted that the answer to unhappiness was to "put one's face on" and never to go out without makeup. She seemed blithely oblivious to my ashen-faced predicament that had gone somewhat beyond making, or masking up. I soon decided I preferred my clothes rumpled.

The final figure in this new group was the psychiatrist. We found him behind a red door set into a tall, Victorian brick terrace, up a narrow flight of stairs fresh-carpeted in

clean, abrasive brown, down a corridor, and through a heavy
fire door.

I always met my new psychiatrist, Dr. B., in the waiting
room. He was very different from Dr. A., introducing himself in a tone of quiet apology. Dr. A. was never keen on dialogue, and once I was off her books she would not see me
unless I was referred by my GP. She had, in practice, a narrow
account to give of postpartum depression. But she had wit,
she was intelligent, and she seemed to give her full attention.
Dr. B. seemed kind, unconcerned, and astonishingly compla-
cent about the dilemma of depression. He talked as though
oblivious of its horror and of how it affects one's life, impli-
cating itself in one's past and one's future. He believed, he
told me, that my depression was an unfortunate physiologi-
cal illness that was fortunately easily treatable with medication and ECT.

There was nothing else for me to do, so back I went to
the shock merchants. When it came to it, I had no therapeu-
tic alternative but convulsions. Psychotherapy, for all my interest, did not seem to be available on the National Health
Service. And having talked to a few psychotherapists, it seems
possible that no psychotherapist would have taken me on in
that state anyway. This time I took my shocks as an outpatient. Though my recollection seems to be chiefly of the first
visit, twice a week for four more weeks I was from midnight,
"nil by mouth," that strange phrase used by British hospitals
to indicate that the patient must not eat or drink before the
anaesthetic is administered.

We took Eliza each time to spend the morning with
Chris, a friend in the village. Then Hugh, Jesse, and I set out

for another hospital. This second hospital looked as forgotten and leftover as its patients. We waited in a dayroom, seated together on a collapsed sofa, for somebody to take me away. The colors of the furniture had got lost long ago. At the back of the room was a large bookcase with old, forgotten books and magazines.

A cheery nurse came for me and we walked down the inevitable long, insipid green corridor. The nurse wore a certain perfume. It's not an unpleasant one, but its smell conjures me back to that corridor walk in a second. There were a few others with us, like the thin girl whose hands and arms were criss-crossed by scabs and scars in neat lines one time, bandaged from palm to elbow another. That day, Hugh says, all the other patients had their arms bandaged too, as though slashing had spread through the ward like an infection.

There was no carpeted ECT suite in this place. We waited in a room like a classroom, with blackboard, tables, and chairs. Leftover props from some forgotten dramatic affair were heaped around the edge, a large, tottering cardboard palm tree leaning from one corner into the room. Then, one by one, we were conducted across the corridor by the cheery nurse and straight into the ECT room. Afterward we were all taken back to a large dining room for tea and toast. Plastic bread and pink jam and more cheeriness. I was relieved I could return to Hugh and my baby, that I didn't have to stay there.

It was a relief to meet her again, drinking tea in
the canteen with the other three or four patients

back from the treatment, all pale and shocked
looking, all with bandaged arms from self-inflicted
wounds like Finn's. She looked shaken and hu-
miliated, disoriented and far away, bearing the
twin scar-like marks on her brow like temporary
stigmata, the only visible sign of the psychiatric
operation she had undergone once more in that
colorless operating theatre that still bore all the
signs of its origin as a Victorian workhouse. We
would flee the building as fast as decently possible.

In these months after Christmas I know, from the diary
Hugh filled in, that people came to stay, family and friends, and
we visited others. But there are no names, places, or events in
my mind. It's empty. I know nothing of the brush and touch
of my days with Hugh, Eliza, and Jesse, not a single breakfast,
story, bathtime, tantrum, diaper change, or cuddle. I remember
none of the times Hugh held me, stopped me from flying into
pieces day after day, none of the countless meals he cooked,
none of his consolation. My gratitude has to be blind, frus-
trating to me and to him.

Toward the end of February, just after I had taken my last
shock, we went out for supper twice. I can still see the green-
ness of Nicole's plants and the whiteness of Joe's walls. This
whiteness spread itself in my memory, for, driving home that
night, we got stuck in a snowdrift a quarter of a mile outside
our village. We walked back through deep snow, Eliza and
Jesse wrapped inside our coats.

Early in March, Eliza had a second birthday party, but I
don't recall it. I did visit Susie, a friend about to give birth to

twins. It took some doing, because the maternity ward of the district hospital was only spitting distance from the Mother and Baby Unit and I had palpitations walking so near. Later in March I went to London to meet my sister, returned after a year away. There was a family wedding and I made marmalade in my mother's kitchen. Though I can name names, there's no texture, no grain to my memory. It's all without affect. For six months or more, it's all like this, as though the substance has been taken out of my recollections and I'm left only with the skeleton.

After Easter Hugh began to return to his work and I to map my daily life with the children. To survive my inner weather I had to focus on the outer weather. Together with Hugh, I evolved a life that I could bear living, just. I had to become the things I'd been fleeing for months: a pragmatist and a "manager." So for months, right into deep summer, the scope of my demand went no further than the doorstep — washing the kitchen floor, doing the ironing, or cooking a meal was the goal for the day. To accomplish that one thing was a vindication of my rediscovered, perhaps reinvented, autonomy, even if the nature of that thing interested me not one whit. It was a convalescence like any other, with good and bad weeks and days.

Sometimes I couldn't manage it all and the terrible inner weather that was always brooding just under my skin exploded. Electrical storms, thunder and hail, or endless rain, seemed to fill the air around me. And I would scream at the children, throw furniture and weep. Then find myself racked with contrition and apologize and try to compensate them for the kind of behavior I'm terrified of receiving myself.

Like all the other women I've talked to who despaired after childbirth, my home in those months was no sanctuary, but a place to be feared. So I took flight from it whenever possible, visiting myself upon friends in every state of mind. Though I could rarely bring myself to say much about what had gone on, they offered me practical solace and never told me to pull myself together. Somehow, when I was out visiting, I was safer from visitation by my own state of mind.

I finished with Dr. B. in the spring but carried on with the antidepressants, as advised, until the following autumn. Summer was a boon time — I had broken the back of the breakdown, so I thought. I'd slumped a little each time I phased down my drugs, but only for a day or two. So stepping lightly out of a summer, which I can't remember, into autumn, I stopped taking the last daily pill a year after Jesse's birth. My depression reawakened immediately, as though from some long torpor. It wasn't the same rage of self-loathing that had sent me into hospital a year earlier. But it was debilitating and at times I've not known how to bear it.

I never considered resuming the pills. They would simply have delayed the dilemma. They enabled me to survive an impossible crisis and helped me compose myself sufficiently to begin life again. But they had no answers for me and they hadn't erased the questions. Like the pelican, I started plucking the flesh from my breast once again, not to feed my young but to feed my self-contempt. Nevertheless, that autumn I was no longer as mesmerized by my own survival as I had been even three months earlier. Now my natural curiosity, squashed beneath all else for a year, began to reassert itself.

> *When we met, she would often appear with*
> *wounds on the back of her hands and on her fore-*
> *head. She did not refer to these and was clearly*
> *embarrassed to have them observed. For a long*
> *time, during my visits, her face would be collapsed*
> *into a shroud of woe, and only very rarely would*
> *it light up with the bright, strong, intelligent smile*
> *I most associate with her.*

Jesse took her first steps when she was a year old. Her early ventures into the pedestrian world run parallel with my efforts to understand what might have happened to me. I took out the questions that had run around my head for a year and gave them some air. The psychiatric treatment had left me with no resources with which to understand or re-solve my intermittent but frightening melancholia. I couldn't remember much of what had gone on in the year, but I had to construct some kind of understanding somehow. So I tried to make an appointment with Dr. A. I wanted to ask her questions: how did she understand postpartum depression, what did she think ECT did, and how did the drugs work? What was the prognosis like if I were to have another child (something I was keen then to do soon) and how long should I wait before doing so? I was curious to know how she would describe the state of mind I was still suffering under. But she refused to see me, unless referred by my GP. This was a blow. Even though she was overworked, etc. like all doctors, I was dismayed that she'd concede no human connection. It wasn't that I wanted treating. I wanted to understand the treatment.

Instead I went to see Dr. B., who saw me willingly. Though I brandished my list of questions, I still failed to penetrate his calm manner. When I asked him what he knew of the effects of ECT on the patient's memory, he suggested I should be relieved to remember so little. He saw no reason to delay having another child. After all, I'd got better the first time, I'd get better again. If the depression struck again, it'd simply be a question of more drugs and more ECT. He failed to see why ECT was disturbing. I failed to ask him whether he'd experienced it himself, to be so blithe. I did manage to say that having an electric shock put through one's skull while unconscious was a distressing experience, but I don't think he chose to think that was important.

When I asked Dr. B. to refer me to a psychologist or psychotherapist, as I knew I had a right to, he asked me to explain, in five minutes, exactly why I thought I needed psychotherapy. I tried to do so, citing my father, but clearly I would have needed a more histrionic narrative to convince him of much. He would refer me, he said, but as I wasn't an urgent case, it might take months for an appointment to come through. I left in a state of fury. Dr. B. had been nice. He'd given me as much time as I wanted. But he refused to acknowledge that my depression had any consequences or part in my life.

A support group met every month at the hospital. So far I'd thrown each reminder in the trash. But one Monday evening in early October, a year after Jesse's birth, I returned to the place, my heart racing. As I walked the long corridor, I was possessed by an anxiety. Like someone returning to their old school, I wondered, all of a sudden, whether I had really graduated from this place at all. It exerted a morbid pull upon me that lasted for days. I found myself yearning to return to that place of my dread.

The ward had been redecorated in my absence, but nothing was changed by that. It felt as uninhabited and bleak as when I had first walked in. I arrived slightly early and entered the empty nursery. No depressed mothers at large, it seemed. As I looked out of the large nursery window, I was looking at a view I'd never seen before. Of course the ECT might have effaced it, but I had no recollection of the small back garden with its neat, autumnal vegetables that I now saw. At that moment the dark patch of earth outside carried the shape of my curiosity, suspended for nearly a year and just daring to return.

The other stories I heard there were as different from my own as the lives of the women who told them. Some had experienced extraordinary delusions, seeing ghouls and goblins, monsters and angels. They remembered shaping the world into bizarre forms, animating ordinary objects like beds, crockery, pills, and food, or imbuing them with far-fetched profundity. Others, more like me, had been struck with appalling self-contempt and the wish to flee their own lives. One woman arrived in a wheelchair, her blue-bruised and swollen legs pinned and spliced with metal because she'd jumped off a motorway bridge a year after her son was born.

Some had left the hospital three years previously and one woman was just about to leave, having been hospitalized for six months. All, except me, were still taking antidepressants. No one felt free from their illness and all were bewildered, with no way of describing or understanding what had happened. Everyone felt guilty, as though the nightmare they had survived was their own responsibility. For many this guilt was affirmed by their partners, who blamed them for their distress.

None of the nurses who organized the group was willing to offer any opinions about the causes, treatment or recovery from postpartum depression. They seemed unsure of the point of the group, expecting the women to know what it was they were coming for. Since all the women, myself included, were in varying states of confusion, embarrassment, and anxiety about what had happened, no one was in a position to do this. I returned for several months out of anger and because I needed to ask questions. Since I failed to vent my anger, couldn't get answers to my questions, and found my support elsewhere, eventually I stopped going.

❖　　❖　　❖

In early November I stopped eating during the day. I just didn't *want* to anymore. It was a conscious decision, but not one I could explain. Jesse and I had just quit breast-feeding, so my body was my own again. I could starve myself without depriving my child. My abstinence was a dry passion I pursued with ferocity. Other people's anxiety only fed my resolve.

As long as I fed my children, I fasted. I turned my stomach from breakfast, lunch, and tea, allowing myself not so much as an apple or a dry piece of bread. It's exhausting, fueling a protest with hunger. The half hour I could steal in the day, with Jesse napping and Eliza watching television, was often consumed by sleep. As I bathed them and got them ready for bed, my fatigue rising by the minute, I waited for Hugh's return. By seven in the evening my limbs ached with my triumph over appetite. As Eliza and Jesse snuggled next to him on the sofa for their bedtime story, I poured a drink and fetched in a bowl of peanuts and my own book. Then, seated opposite, I gave myself up to utter self-absorption, momentarily a spectator of my children's lives. I can still taste the intoxication of that first nut, its very saltiness the signal to my stomach that help was at hand. Once the kids were in bed, Hugh and I would cook and eat an evening meal.

After two months of this I had lost roughly twenty-eight pounds and looked too thin. I was worried that my weight loss would prevent me from leading my life but I was powerless to start eating. Perhaps a well-timed "threat," of sectioning or ECT was all that was needed. I don't think so. I needed to empty myself and this was the only way I knew how. Not eating was a way of keeping something at bay, just.

Lunchtime was awkward, if I was eating with other adults too. Occasionally I'd eat a couple of mouthfuls, for the sake of appearances. It made me feel awful, self-contemptuous, displaced into some shadowland of identity. It wasn't long before I started making myself sick, even if I'd eaten only a tiny amount. I couldn't bear to keep the food inside me.

My behavior was like a body-blow to Hugh. I felt like I'd punched him in the stomach. He didn't want to ask friends to supper because mealtimes had become a trial, not a feast, for him. He became worried, sometimes angry. At first I couldn't bear to talk about it, as though I had to barricade my words into my shrinking body. When I did, it made no difference. Surely somewhere in my childhood or adolescence I could find some bit of explanation. Or in my life as a mother, or as a woman without a cause. We found connections and explanations, but I didn't start to eat.

At my wits' end, my own self-starvation drove me into a conversation I'd always promised myself I'd have when I was very rich. I could see that getting psychotherapy on the NHS might never happen, or not for months. And when it did, it'd be a very limited strike operation. So I decided to go for it privately. I'd tried the psychiatrists, the support group, my friends, and the patience of my husband. I didn't know where else to turn and I was getting desperate.

I was living in the world now, looking after my children, playing with them, enjoying and being infuriated by them. Not only could I "keep house" again, but I was determined to resume my intellectual life. I was to edit *Jane Eyre* for a publisher. It seemed apt that I should be working on a story with a madwoman up in its attic. After all, I was my own Bertha Mason, using my body as a whipping-boy for something I couldn't bear to name. In the thick of all my competence, I still nourished myself on hunger and the same raw pain that had burst from me a year ago. I'd started denting the wall again, and drawing blood with my nails from the shocked whiteness on my hands and face.

I'd reached a cul-de-sac. I'd survived the breakdown, I was off the drugs. But I had nothing to say for myself and was hard-pressed to treat myself kindly. Though friends were congratulating me on the speed of my return to ordinary

life, I knew that my daily hunger was a protest against something I still couldn't countenance. And I didn't know any
way out of the impasse. Powerless as ever to describe what I
felt, in late November I visited a psychotherapist to try to
do just that. I've always had a taste for talk. So psychotherapy, in that sense, seemed right up my alley.

He listened hard, sitting in a chair across from me, and
made a few compelling remarks. But he would see me a
minimum of three times a week, financially impossible to
contemplate. He recommended someone else to me and I
visited her in early December. She, too, seemed to listen hard
and make the occasional, intelligent interjection. Enough
was enough and we made a date to begin in January.

It seems appropriate that I have been paying for this psychotherapy with money left me by my grandmother. After
all, my depression has been, in part, a result of my family history. Now that the money is gone, we have a lodger at the
end of our long cottage. Her rent buys me my two analytic
hours. It's odd how uncomfortable people seem to be when
they find out that I drive a thirty-five-mile round trip twice
a week just to talk about myself for fifty minutes, and then
pay for it.

What I do with my grandmother's legacy can't change
what has gone on, but it's given me different stories to tell
by way of understanding. Though I still don't know what to
make of it all, I can see how my recent horror is tied up tight
to the life I am constructed within. Given how much I like
fooling about with words, it was inevitable that my next step
should be to write about it all, the life and the horror.

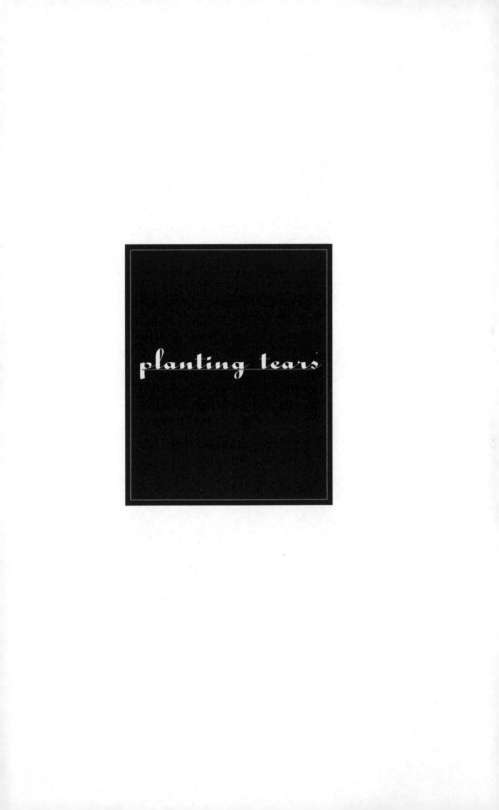

planting tears

WHEN I WAS A LITTLE GIRL, I always had my suitcase packed, so my mother told me. If the word came down that I was off visiting, my bag would be filled up in a moment, ever so neatly. Inside that dark dry place, all my different needs could be squashed reassuringly against one another, toothbrush folded into the crease of my trousers, book nestling in the armpit of a sweater. Living between parents, I carried my home on my back, like the snail.

The best present I ever had from my dad was a floppy blue suitcase with green piping. When it wasn't going anywhere, it squashed into a tiny bundle and tucked into the corner of a drawer. But I could shake it out into something capacious, capable of carrying all I could wish from one place to another. Though my bags have changed since then, their imaginary baggage hasn't.

Not long ago I went to London for the weekend to see friends and then spent Monday visiting people in London about this book. I took counsel about my heavy, red bag. "Check it in the Left Luggage at King's Cross first thing," I was advised, "so you can travel light." The day had enough of a weight of worries as it was. But what happened? The subway stopped at King's Cross and I stayed on. So from half past eight in the morning until six in the evening I carried with me this demon of a thing from one side of London to another, the strap marking a channel across my shoulder. What on earth was in it that I couldn't let it go?

It certainly contained more than my underwear and a pair of jeans. There was this manuscript at the top, for one, its words finding their ballast in my past. But among the books and shoes I'd also dumped the other lives not told, those I'd had to choose against. That day, each time I met another stranger, they commiserated with me upon my load, no more realizing than I that I needed them to see it. They must see that what I had written and shown them was by no means the only story I had.

By lunchtime I'd reached Bayswater. It was half past twelve and my meeting was at one. Banging hips with others as we climbed from the subway, I contemplated the next thirty minutes. There was window-shopping in Whiteleys or reading in the park. But instead I toted my aching shoulder down Queensway, right, then right again. As I walked my eye caught on the buildings to left and right. Like playing a skipping game learned as a child, my glance moved, at first unsurely and then with its own remembered rhythm. It was all there, the tatty high-rises, the traffic island, and the smart mansion flats; even the barbed wire around the painted playground looked the same. The paint was peeling from the house we lived in twenty-five years ago and nobody in the row had a doormat outside any more. I supposed they'd get stolen. I'd lived half a life here until I was six years old and hadn't walked this way since then. Now I'd returned, just for a moment, with another kind of house on my back.

The art of memory is the art of making connections. How to make sense of what often seem like random recollections; how to organize them so they add up to the person I envisage myself as now. My breakdown had been like a collision with an iceberg. I knew from the start it was only the tip. Reaching deep into the opaque blue water of memory, I wanted to find a shape beneath, something of the vast mass underpinning that depression. At first with each plunge, my fingers, tapping in the words, seemed to touch a different random fragment. Gradually these resolved themselves into something solid, a single piece. It floats too deep for my blind fingers to brush it all, but I have, at least, found a body beneath my recent past.

Before I began to write, discovering the joints between my recent misery and my life seemed to involve more artifice than art. But writing uncovers connections the writer was never aware of. And relying on this, I will end this preamble that can amble nowhere till I tell the other parts of this story.

Not long ago I discovered myself weeping as I listened to an Irish nineteenth-century ballad. The refrain went, "Hold me now, O hold me now / Till the hour has gone around / And I'm off on the rising tide / For to face Van Diemen's Land." I was possessed by something, but it wasn't the appalling fate of the Irishmen for whom the song was written. It was the memory of my own leavetaking, as I felt it at that moment, dragged unwilling from my father's arms. The song conjured up to me the desolation I felt when my stay with him was over and I had to say goodbye. It was something that began when I was two or so and ended only with his death, when I was twenty.

I'm sure I've inhabited different shapes at different times. But there's been another, consistent secret life running inside all of them. My public life as a child, from the age of three, was a stable, relatively affluent one with loving parents, beloved and rivalrous younger sisters, and plenty of friends. There were serious hiatuses in this, of course, but no more than beset most children. By the time I was eleven I had been bullied for a season, flashed at, like all London girls, had fights with best friends, and failed to get into the school I was destined for. But I was happy. In a way the story was the same at eighteen. After a successful school career, with lots of sports, lots of study, some good friends, no sex (I was too religious by then), and more periods of painful and mysterious bullying, I was off to the university and leaving home. I was a well-adjusted, intelligent, middle-class girl.

Then there was my secret life. My parents had divorced when I was very young and I lived for most of my childhood with my mother, stepfather John, and two sisters, Jules and Lucy, from this second marriage. I visited my father fairly regularly, in London, Somerset, Oxfordshire, and Kent, as he moved jobs about the country. For my first years' visiting, he lived with a girlfriend I adored called Gina. Then, when I was about seven, he married Tricia. She, too, had been married before and had three children. Richard and Martin stood on either side of me in age, Sylvie was a few years younger. When I was ten Dad and Tricia had their own son, Michael. Moving between my two families was to move between two lives.

My mother vowed never to criticize my father to me, as far as she could help it. This decision to stay silent has always been seen as a piece of heroic and correct self-sacrifice, by me as well as by my family and friends. And she kept to it until he died. But it also licensed a refusal on her part. She would never talk of him to me, as though by not speaking of him he was no longer there. I learned nothing of their life together, good or bad. The refusal went still further. She never really wanted to know what my life with him was like. She tolerated my chat when I returned from a visit, but she'd make no effort of imagination so as to talk with me. It was, and still is, as though the wounds she received while with him were still open. She could bear no pressure on them and, to shut me up, often assumed a mantle of boredom when I wanted to tell her all about his world. She needed to excise him from her life and couldn't bear that he was part of mine.

My sisters were curious about this other place I went to, but always seemed somewhat incredulous. As if amazed that I could countenance another family elsewhere, like some kind of guilty secret. As though I had a choice. They were happiest when able to disparage. When my brothers behaved badly or got into trouble, or I returned with stories of being teased, or unhappy, my sisters wanted to know. Otherwise they, too, were unable to rouse much interest. Though uncomfortable with the notion of ambivalent feelings, my stepfather was the most straightforwardly curious to know. So it was often to him I'd talk about my dad. The effect of this familial refusal was to leave me with a sense that this part of my life, so important to me, was not interesting to anyone else.

This also happened the other way around, providing a curious equilibrium. My father and that family assumed, when I arrived to see them, that I would drop all the baggage of my other life and simply fit in. I don't think it occurred to them that I found it so hard to jump between lives. I've never been able to check my bags. Everything was done differently, of course, and that was also what I liked. I liked and hated the ambivalence of being two daughters in two families, with different jokes, teasing, food, games, kinds of privacy, and so on.

I have a few images of life with Mum between husbands, nothing from earlier on. Whatever I know of that first place has become displaced — or replaced — elsewhere. Before she married John, I recall sharing a small, narrow room for a while, her bed near the door and my cot near the window, end-to-end. And being read *Babar* in bed by one of her roommates. At about the same age, I lay down one evening to sleep on a camp bed in John's bachelor flat. I'd been placed in the dining room. To the left, above me, was a vast, dark-wooded, glass-fronted bookcase. I could just make out the shapes of the objects behind the shiny glaze. This cliff of a thing, reaching high above me, had me mesmerized with fear. It never occurred to me to call out to my mother.

From the age of one, while my mother worked, I attended a day nursery. Once my parents were estranged, the theory was that Dad would pay the nursery fees, and Mum everything else. The practice, no surprise, was that when Dad stopped paying the fee reliably, Mum paid instead. She preferred doing this rather than involving herself in more negotiations with the man she'd determined to be done with.

We ate lunch downstairs in the nursery. We were told that if anyone could eat their pea soup without being sick, they'd get a lollipop. It sounds an improbable bribe to present to a two-year-old, but adults do say improbable things to children. Each Wednesday I spent the evening and night with Jessica, one of the nannies. She had a flat above the nursery. I used to sit in her armchair, in my dressing gown, watching *Batman* on the television at six o'clock as a special treat. I cannot find my father anywhere at this time, though I gather that I saw him quite regularly, because, like us, he lived in London when I was very small.

Trying to piece together the shape of my first years is impossible in the face of my mother's deliberate lack of memory. She still cannot bear to look back before her second marriage. Except for Mum saying I was lonely as a little girl, I don't know what I was like as a toddler. My stepfather, a great tease, tells me I was a sulky little girl when he first met me (and the implication is often that I haven't changed). I was given to temper tantrums and it's agreed I was a "difficult" child. But then I was in a "difficult," if common, situation.

On the day of my mother's second marriage, I cycled my trike around outside the house. I didn't go to the ceremony, because they thought I would be too much to handle. Later I was distracted by one of their friends playing a rough-and-tumble game, leaving Mum and John free to escape for their honeymoon. My maternal grannie, whom I adored, came up to London from Devon to stay with me for the two weeks.

John took me on as his own daughter as far as that was possible. I was not his own, and the fact never escaped me. I have been asked whether I ever thought of calling him Daddy. The question has never made sense to me. I had a daddy, whom I visited. I couldn't have two. When I wanted to upset John, I am told I used to say, "You're only treating me like this because you're my stepfather." John is a fine jazz pianist and the cruelest act I could commit, when about three, was to hunch up at the furthest point in the room and tell him, "I'll sit in the corner and I won't even listen." As though somehow I could shut him out. Later, we developed a jokey, genial, prickly relationship, in which he usually referred to himself as the "Wicked Stepfather." This was a joke of course, so far-fetched as to be ridiculous. Nevertheless it did give a ritual place to the difference, always played down and always present, between me and his blood children, my sisters.

Mum wanted to have a child with John as soon as possible after they were married. It was important to her to show that this new marriage, which had made her happy, had replaced the old, disastrous one. But for me, the product of, and unavoidable testimony to, the old one, this can't have been so easy. I imagine that the usual fears of the oldest child must have been compounded by some sense that I represented something my mother wanted to replace. My sister was born at home when I was four, thirteen months after the marriage. I remember that day. One neighbor had told me to come and tell her as soon as the baby arrived and I did so. I jumped from one doormat to the next, a popular game along the modern terrace of houses we lived in, and rang the neighbor's doorbell. She was delighted to see me, and if she was annoyed at being woken at seven, a little early on a Sunday, she certainly didn't show it. I traveled these same doormats when, on another occasion, I announced I was leaving home, again in my nightie. I didn't get beyond the last one before returning, humiliated by my failure to escape.

My second sister was born twenty-two months after my first, and the family was complete. I think I lived an ostensibly happy life as a small child. My mother had more time to give to her family now that she didn't have to go out to work, and she loved us all thoroughly. She says she was never very good at playing with us when we were small and envies my capacity to play with Eliza and Jesse. Maybe it's because she's not that interested in the world children inhabit and doesn't stop for long to listen. Perhaps back then she was too engrossed, first by her unhappiness with my father, and then by her happiness with John, to give much of an ear.

We were well-off, able to have most of what we wanted, with au pairs to boot, some of whom I loved and some not. I loved my sisters and played with them; my relationship with John developed into something remarkable, given the circumstances conspiring around it. And I visited my father

regularly, visits organized mainly by my mother. But somewhere at the heart of all this, I felt I was not listened to.
Possibly the kind of conversation, or attention, I needed was
something my mother couldn't bear to give me. With so
much emphasis on this game of "happy families," I was left
no room to think differently. The party line, which I
heeded, was always, "What an impressive family, and he's not
even her real father."

❖   ❖   ❖

Since my father died I have faced what seems an impossible
task. For ten years I've been in search of the right memories. What I long to recall are the times I had my father to
myself. Just me and him. Now that I think about it, the task
began way before he died. I have a few images framed and
set high on a shelf in my mind. When I was perhaps five I
remember us watching a Western on television, eating sar-
dines on toast, seated together in a big armchair. A few years
later when I was about eight I was in a car crash with him.
Not only was he accident-prone, but he was also a terrible
driver, aggressive and speedy. I saw the accident shape itself
in the seconds before it happened, as I offered my dad a
peanut from the back seat. It was in the fast lane of the highway and the car was a write-off. We were both more or less
unhurt. We got a lift to the nearest train station in a truck.
Squashed in the cab between my father and the truck driver in a fug of shock and sleepiness, I was perfectly happy.
When we arrived at my father's house, my stepmother, concerned, asked whether I was all right. My shoulder hurt

quite badly, but I said I was fine, already anxious not to be thought of as plaintive and wanting the impossible — to seem as tough as my stepbrothers.

Once Dad had remarried, I rarely had him to myself. I hated sharing him. Though I got on well with my stepbrothers, I resented their intimacy with my father. It was something I was desperate for and couldn't grasp. I was very close to my mother, but I knew I had her love. My love for him was like a guilty secret. I could tell nobody else about it.

My father was a charmer. He seemed a little like Peter Pan, endlessly in flight from the very thing he wanted most. And women, including his daughter, suffered the consequences of this impossible journey. I found it impossible not to adore him, but equally impossible to know him. He was exasperatingly absent, but apparently oblivious to this. When I beat a retreat, fearful of being ignored by this man I loved but didn't understand, he was upset. It didn't seem to occur to him that there was anything problematic in our relationship at all. There is no doubt that I became a sulky teenager, but he was an even sulkier adult.

Dad always wanted a son. So my mother told me after he had died. When I was ten he had one, though I didn't hear of it for a while. Whether Michael satisfied him in the way I couldn't, I don't know. I suspect his wishes were beyond satisfaction. My stepbrothers, so close to me in age, became sons of a kind to him. Though I was an effective tomboy, I couldn't compete with them. I was tall and athletic and as robust as I knew how, but however far I could throw, they could throw further; however fast I could ride my bike, they could ride faster. They could run quicker, dig deeper, and lift more. So in the end I withdrew. I refused to compete and my father, oblivious to the root of my misery, used to berate me. Once again I was the sulky little girl. I don't know what he expected of me, but unable to provide it, his rage obviously proved more bearable to me than his disappointment.

When I want to conjure up my father, I often return in my mind's eye to a small island in a loch off the west coast of Scotland. It was a place close to my father's heart. I traveled there with him and what I find myself calling *his* family for three or four summers. We stayed in a small wooden cabin, gathering water from a spring five minutes' walk away, cooking on a small gas stove, and slipping on drenched ferns in the rain on the way to the outdoor privy at night. We, the children, spent the days making expeditions around the island, helping the farmers dip the sheep that grazed the island and building elaborate dens in the bracken. There were hills to climb and freezing clear water in which to fish, canoe, and swim. We explored rock pools and played long games on the deserted hulk of an old landing craft at the far end of our magic beach. I loved the remote, beautiful, bleak landscape. It was easier to be in my father's family here, away from all homes. A formidably unreliable man, he seemed to find the notion of being only in one place, of having one home, unbearable. He'd never had a reliable one as a child and adulthood seemed an impossible place to start. As I was to discover after he died, he left a litany of other lives, each unknown to the other. But on the small island in the remote sea loch he seemed able to tolerate the idea of his own presence. At least that's how I remember it.

Sometimes the unfamiliarity of this family of mine felt like too much to bear, so far from anywhere else. I didn't get the jokes, or I didn't want to join in, or I wanted to slip off and read. Or I was too greedy, or too fastidious. I remember a hot day and the discovery of a beautiful beach at the far end of the island. We wanted to swim. Someone suggested swimming naked. There was no one around for miles. Everyone else, robustly unembarrassed, took their clothes off. I was about fourteen and excruciatingly ashamed. I didn't want them to see my naked body. I didn't let anybody see it. Perhaps they thought it was good for me to face out my embarrassment, but I was made to undress. As the warm air stroked my thighs and stomach, breasts and bottom, I loathed my womanliness and wished there was nothing there to see. On another occasion I was down by the boat with my father and brothers. Martin had dropped a key, by mistake, over the side of the boat, into deep water. So Dad stripped off all his clothes to dive and retrieve it. I was profoundly ill at ease and my brothers teased me, telling me I was gawking at my father's prick. Maybe I was. I never saw men naked. But I denied it, dismayed again by my incapacity to fit in and feel as I felt I was meant to. Neither of my families was going to make room for the other and I wanted to be in both.

My brothers teased me often and I dare say I was as sullen and awkward to them at times as they were rude and difficult to me. But on one particular holiday they bullied me and then it was frightening, feeling absolutely on the outside. I had joined my father's family for a holiday in Thurlestone, Devon. They were staying with family friends who had a house there. My brothers and sister ganged up against me, together with the three children in the other family. I had a small room to myself on the ground floor and I locked the door when I went to bed. Even so, I was terrified they would find a way in through the window. I used to weep when I went to bed. As a butt for their malice, the more upset I became, the more it spurred them on. It was as though, just for that week, my brothers were free to see me as somebody to be mocked, so far on the outside of everything. My other family remembers me returning in a state of trauma. I was anxious that nothing be said to my dad or stepmother because it would confirm all their worst thoughts about me and next time I saw them things would be more difficult. I never saw the other family again as a child and my brothers never repeated that kind of bullying. But from then on I felt like an endangered species in that family. My status was so precarious that I could be displaced into the void by any outsider. I held on to my place with tenterhooks.

When I was twelve my mother asked if I would like to make the arrangements to see my dad. I was delighted, for it seemed to me a symbol of my maturity. She also stopped reminding him of my birthday or of Christmas approaching. The first time he forgot my birthday I was devastated. Not even a card. And I soon discovered that his promises were like water. If he said he'd phone back, he never did. Of course I persevered because I had to see him. My mother had never hinted of the difficulties that existed in the face of my father's compulsive unreliability. I learned to make arrangements with Tricia rather than Dad, and she, I think, was responsible for the presents remembered in the years to Dad's death. He never failed to collect me for a visit if he had promised to do so, but he was always late. Nevertheless those journeys were treasures to me. I had him to myself. On one occasion he stopped the car and we hugged one another. It only happened once and I hold the memory to me as passionately as I once wrapped my arms around my father's middle.

My first school was a big London primary school. Here I thrived as one of the boys. It had one of those extraordinarily antisocial playgrounds of blacktop, much of it on a slope. I incurred the injuries appropriate to such a playing surface, taking home gravel beneath my knee each week. But I bore my war wounds heroically and with pride. They confirmed that I was part of the action. When I was seven we moved house and I to a new school. This one was still run in a sit-up-and-beg manner. We sat behind desks and the playground was segregated, girls from boys. Only during kiss-chase did children run the gauntlet of the teachers' wrath and cross the thin white line. I always felt too much an outsider to join in these playground games. Perhaps I didn't want to be one of the girls. Here I was bullied by an older child, an enormous girl without a face in my mind. Again and again I'd arrive home in tears but never tell why. At my third school I felt at home and I thrived for the three years I was there. My report says I was even good at math. I took delight in organizing my playground gang. I was popular, at the hub of the action, brushing off accusations of corruption unperturbed.

High school was another world. I arrived into a class of thirty girls, about half of whom had been at the junior high. They had decided for good reasons to punish the new ones.

They would have nothing to do with us, not speaking to us even if we addressed them. I was already disoriented and vulnerable in this huge place. There were no children's pictures on the walls, and it had strange bells and rhythms. Grown-up girls wearing bras beneath white shirts and ties strode down the corridors and the teachers didn't smile. Being ostracized made life hell for a while. Eventually, after perhaps six weeks, I broke the back of the silence because I could play games. Not mind games but outdoor ones. I was selected as defense reserve for a Saturday netball game and my class esteem rocketed.

Puberty was reviled in my class at school. Not by everyone, but by those who held the balance of power. These girls were, no coincidence, the slowest to develop breasts and pubic hair and the last to start their periods. I felt humiliated because I had my first period at age twelve and I was already full-breasted at fourteen. During swimming lessons, the girls with no pubic hair strutted their lack of stuff while we others tried to hide the dark patch at the groin that appeared when our swimsuits were wet. For a while I used to pluck out my pubic hair with a pair of tweezers. Futility, rather than any pleasure in the hair, made me give this up.

Our sports teacher joined in the humiliation game. After playing games outdoors, we had to run through the cold communal shower before putting our school clothes back on. This teacher would take the towels from the pegs and heap them on the floor in a mass of tangled colors so that everyone had to scrimmage for their own. Snug in her sweatsuit, she laughed at the girls who, with breasts swinging, searched frantically through the pile for their privacy.

Netball was played seriously at my school and no one was more serious in their play than I. I loved the drip and exhaustion of training, the complicity of the team. I gave up weekends and evenings happily to matches and tournaments. My school team was very good. Then, when I was about fifteen, I made it into the junior county squad. That meant a subway ride to Paddington with my best friend every Tuesday after school. Together with about twenty-five other teenage girls, we ran around the Edgware Road in short skirts and worked out through the winter months under an amber floodlit glow. There I was harangued — to jump higher, run faster, or be better — to my heart's content. I was never good enough to keep pace with my friend to the top, but I wore the Middlesex county colors on weekends regularly for a while and shouted out with gusto against Surrey, Wiltshire, Notts, Sussex, and Devon.

I was never quite at ease among the Middlesex netball players. Too keen to belong, I played in fear of disparagement and rejection. I've invented many female coteries since then to which I'm never fully admitted, but this group of sweaty women was the first. The needy search for friends with bosoms must have begun at home. My sisters' closeness to one another has always left me feeling something of an honorary, rather than a necessary, member of the sisterhood. Not quite fully paid up. Until recently I always felt no woman could really think me important enough to have as a friend. At times I still wonder why they do.

I've always wanted to write something special. At secondary school this desire soon became entangled with a passionate admiration for my English teacher. But my efforts to write and please Miss Davis received very mediocre marks for the first couple of years. Then one weekend I wrote an essay that I knew was different from anything I had done before. I can recall only the bones of it, but the impression that inspired it is still sharp in my mind.

One Sunday evening, driving home with a friend and her family from an excursion, I had seen a house on fire. We were in a traffic jam somewhere in south London and passed the burning building across the street very slowly. The house seemed already partly collapsed. On one side I could see the wallpaper and fireplaces of rooms no longer there. Standing on the pavement was a family. Both parents were cradling small children. A third child stood beside them in her nightie, watching her home burn. It seemed terrible that she should be outside in the wrong clothes, unable to change them. I knew I had found the words to say something I needed to. When the essay got a better mark than anything I had written before, it was a vindication of something I already knew I'd done.

The supernatural terrifies me beyond endurance; I can't stomach it. But the only other essay I remember from my childhood was about exactly the kind of inchoate fear I am most afraid of. This time I used a story told me by a family friend. A friend of hers called Jane had gone to see a house for sale, taking her dog with her. The house was empty and she had a key from the real estate agent. As she walked up the garden path to the front door the dog, uncharacteristically, started whining. He was unwilling to go through the front door. She walked around the downstairs rooms and he continued to moan. He wouldn't follow her upstairs so, slightly disconcerted, she climbed the staircase alone. She entered one of the bedrooms and was struck with horror. There was nothing in there, but she fled.

When Jane returned the key with this story, the real estate agent told her that an awful murder had been committed in that particular room. So the only stories I remember writing describe the home as a particular kind of nightmare, even though in the main I am like the woman's dog. I flee at the faintest whiff from any tales of terrible defamiliarization.

❖   ❖   ❖

When I was about nine, I saw the madwoman in the attic for the first time. *Jane Eyre* was being serialized on TV and a babysitter allowed me to stay up late and watch it. She wasn't interested, so I sat alone on the sofa in my nightie. I watched Bertha Mason come into Jane's room the night before her wedding and tear Jane's wedding veil and I was too frightened to move. I couldn't cross the room and turn the television off, nor could I reach down the other end of the sofa for a cushion to hide my eyes. Like a mouse before a snake, I was mesmerized with fear.

My bedroom was at the top of the house. I liked being up there, in the attic as it were. Everyone else had bedrooms on the floor below. There was a large stair window made of small rectangles of stained glass that you headed toward and then away from as you climbed the stairs. One of the panes had a small hole in it and I became convinced that the madwoman was going to come through that hole and get me. So every night my stepfather, or somebody else, had to stand on the first floor landing and watch me up to my room until, years later, the window was double-glazed and my fear contained.

When I was very young I used to be afraid that a snake was under my bed. Sleep came only if my blankets were over my head. If any part of me, a toe or a hair, was outside the covers or over the edge, the snake would get me. By the time I was seven I had transformed this fear of snakes into a passion for them. I learned all I could about them and loved visiting the reptile house at the London Zoo. For a short while I kept a grass snake I'd found on vacation with a friend in a bathtub in her garden. I liked the dry, smooth touch of its skin and the run of its body. It moved like an athlete at its peak, each part of its length forming part of its motion. It seems that I'm trying to do with my life now what I did with the snake under my bed. Having been afraid of my past, and what I would find there, I'm now involved in a kind of grand passion with it. I want to learn to love the touch of its skin. It's the only skin I have, after all.

A while ago Hugh and I were discussing first novels, and the idea that they were often written quite closely out of childhood. I said I couldn't imagine writing such a thing because I'd always thought of myself as having an uneventful, ordinary, happyish, middle-class childhood. The irony of this remark didn't strike me even as we were having the conversation. On one level that is what I'd always thought.

But I'd never stopped to think — never dared to stop and think — why this supposedly happy girl had done the things she'd done. I'd never brooded on them, nor had I ever spoken about them to anybody else. And for a time even my postpartum breakdown seemed to have come out of the ether, and the grief I felt for my father then seemed to be something separate from the normal condition of my life.

Then, when I began to write about my breakdown and to consider where it might have come from (because in the end I don't believe in ether), my memories gave me a picture of a different kind. For the first time I was trying to imagine why I'd become so unhappy. For the first time my own self-censorship began to crumble. I began to see the holes and insecurities. The apparently confident, sheltered girl had successfully hidden, even from herself, the dark despair that finally brought her world crashing down about her ears years later. The terrifying iceberg of emotions that I have been struck by since Jesse's birth had its deepest parts floating way down out of sight in my own early life.

❖　　❖　　❖

I've always wished I could tell better lies, not thinking of myself as someone very good at it. If I'd seen more of my dad, I've joked, it's an art I would have picked up from him. And yet for years I have embodied a particular lie. But it has lain so deep that it never even occurred to me until very recently that it was one, perhaps because it expressed a truth about my unconscious condition. It was something I was compelled to do, though I never asked myself why. The only thing that seems clear now is that I must have been suffering from a terrible pain, but not one I could acknowledge. So I reinvented it and embodied it. It became written in my body.

My heart races as I write this. It does every time I talk of what seems to me both a terrible lie and an awful truth. When I was twelve I got a bad backache, which was first diagnosed as something like growing pains. I was in the bath when I heard my aunt reassure my concerned mother. It was nothing to worry about, she said, it'd be better in a few days. At that moment I became determined that she would be wrong. It wasn't better in a few days, I dragged it on and on. There were X-rays, doctors, and physiotherapy.

Over the next few years I was regularly incapacitated by pain in my back. I went to a bevy of experts, had tests, more physiotherapy, lost weeks of school, and gained a lot of sympathy and attention from friends, teachers, relatives, even relative strangers. And I had found the secret to endless solicitude and worry from my mother. But I had no back pain. It was an invention. My groans and grimaces, my awkward posture, and my endurance were all fictitious, at least as far as my spine was concerned. I cost my family dear. Maybe I needed to know I was doing just that.

When I was about fourteen I precipitated a crisis. I took to my bed in terrible pain and refused to allow myself to be manipulated out of it. I was beyond physiotherapy, or anything else. After days of agony for my mother and stepfather, I was taken by ambulance to the hospital. It drove, with flashing lights, and at a snail's pace to minimize the jarring on my spine, into London. Admitted immediately, I spent the next nine weeks in there, the summer holidays and more. Our vacation was canceled, my sisters having to make do with day trips here and there. Mum and John visited me every day, trying to leave their fraught expressions outside the door. My father visited me once, with his family. They came at lunchtime while I was not eating a plate of institutional roast beef, two vegetables, and gravy on a tray before me. My dad told me off for not eating my lunch and then ate it himself. When they left, he said he would visit me again the following day, by himself. But he never did. I don't know who he wanted to punish by letting me down like this. Not me necessarily. But it felt like a terrible indictment, as though if I'd been a more compelling daughter, he'd have returned.

I was put in a plaster cast from neck to waist for a few weeks, to see if it would help. While still unused to its weight I rolled over on my bed to reach for a glass of water. The weight of the cast created a momentum that continued the roll and I ended up on the floor, hitting my head on my bedside cupboard on the way. I was taken off for an X ray — a statutory obligation, I was told. While waiting my turn, on my bed with a nurse in attendance, I shut my eyes. And then decided not to open them again. They thought I had blacked out because of the fall. I refused to respond to noises or prods. My bed was moved into a single room and there I remained, apparently unconscious, for about eight hours. Nothing would rouse me. Sharp pins were stuck in my feet, I was talked to, whispered to, suddenly shouted at, appealed to. My reflexes were poor and my pulse dropped worryingly low. A piece was sawn out of the plaster cast in case artificial resuscitation was needed.

I listened to myself being talked of in the third person and it confirmed my dissociation. I felt as though I could leave my inert body behind and draw myself in; remove myself from the matter at hand and play dead for a while. It was a relief. Mum and John were summoned. A neurosurgeon was called in and he whispered in my ear: "If I have to operate on your brain, I'll have to shave all your hair off and then get a drill." His voice went on and on. Soon after this whisper I began to return.

After this, I used to black out regularly, sometimes for half an hour, sometimes for several hours. I was given a brain scan and a psychiatrist came to see me asking questions about my broken home. But no one could find out what was wrong. I didn't know either, but I wish they'd tried harder. Finally my parents were told that all the hospital could conclude was that my body couldn't take the pain, so periodically I took to unconsciousness. This diagnosis was perhaps more right than wrong, even though I was never in fact unconscious. Internally I was running away from something, though I never got away.

Now that I had got as far as hospitalization, nothing worked for the pain. Not bed rest, nor the plaster cast, nor traction, nor painkillers. Unsurprisingly, nothing showed up on the X ray. But the problem was located with another test, which did come as a surprise to me. A milogram was performed after I'd been in the hospital for about five weeks. A dye was injected into my spinal column, I was tipped up and down to flush it around my spine, and then photographed, as it were. My consultant announced that a slipped disc had shown up. And since it seemed utterly recalcitrant to conservative treatment, the only course of action left was to operate. Which is what he did. I didn't worry at any point about being found out, nor about the actual consequences of spinal surgery. After the operation, as I lay in bed experiencing acute (postoperative) pain in my back for the first time, my doctor explained that not only had he had to remove most of the slipped disc — an operation called a laminectomy — but he had discovered what he described as nerves going down the wrong holes. He had set these right. If only it had really been that easy.

I wasn't happy, doing all this. But there didn't seem any other way to go. A balcony skirted my eighth-floor ward and, once I was on my feet, I used to go out and admire the view. It hadn't much drama in it — rooftops, busy roads, a bit of the Thames, and an enormous warehouse with "Harrods Depository" printed on the roof. I was dismayed to learn that a depository was just another name for a warehouse. Standing in the eighth-floor breeze, I wondered, just once, whether it wouldn't be better to jump.

Two weeks after the operation I left the hospital. I'd made a good recovery and walked out thin and institution-alized. I'd stopped eating, more or less, toward the end of my stay. Though I was seduced back to food while still in the hospital by the smell of hot buttered toast, I weighed only 105 pounds when I came home. On my five-foot-ten-inch, big-boned frame, this looked deathly. None of my clothes would stay on me except a pair of overalls, suspended by their straps. I put the weight on quickly once home, unable as ever to resist my mother's food.

Home was terrifying at first. I had to relearn my life. Nothing felt assured. I didn't want to resume the responsi-bilities I'd fled so dramatically two and a half months previ-ously. I wanted to be back in that place where everything was

given to me and nothing asked for in return, not even love
and affection. At home, and inevitably at school, I felt as if I'd
been left behind. It was as though I couldn't, or couldn't bear
to, inhabit the places that were mine. I was miserable, and
inarticulate.

My physical pain, albeit invented, had given me a legitimate trauma. It had entitled me to sympathy that was above
board. Writing this, I am sure that when they read it, those
closest to me during my teenage years will feel they've been
cheated, as though I have tricked them into extremities of
feeling they needn't have experienced. They'll be furious to
have been put through so much unnecessary suffering. The
few people to whom I've told this tale have wondered what
kind of despairing need lived in me that compelled me to
go to such lengths. And I've found it hard to answer them.

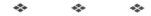

We had a lodger called Kim at home. She lived in a room on
the first floor and she'd become a close friend of mine. She
was religious in a way I'd never encountered before. What
she believed in didn't stop in church, as I'd always assumed
God did. It came home with her. Since I spent hours in her
company, talking, drinking coffee, meeting her friends, I became accustomed to these beliefs, though they weren't mine.

Then one afternoon, several months after leaving the
hospital, I had another terrible argument with my younger
sister Lucy. As often happened at the time, we'd goaded one
another into a fury, though I knew I was right. I went to take
a shower and, closing the bathroom door, I said a prayer: "If

you're there, God, I want a written apology from Lucy as proof." The shower had a glass door. As I stood beneath the gush, through the steamy smear of water I saw a small piece of paper appear, pushed beneath the bathroom door. That apology may have cost nine-year-old Lucy dear. Little did I realize how dear it would cost me.

Soon after meeting Hugh I used to describe myself around a dinner table as "someone who used to be a fundamentalist Christian." Hugh admitted recently he got a little tired of the story. For all he was interested in my experience, he wondered when I was going to allow in other versions of myself.

These days I can't make head or tail of it. Called to account, I mumble. Every time I set about explaining on paper what I believed then, and why, I am sucked, in the instant, within an argot that is like a clashing of cymbals in my ear. It makes no sense, it seems to have nothing to do with who I am now. The system of belief around which I organized most of my teenage life is so dismaying that I have to believe my conversion was a product of something else, some need particular to me as the individual I was at fourteen.

So perhaps it was that it offered a kind of belonging where everyone was equally related. There were no "half" or "step" relations in my church. And presiding over it all was a father figure to end all father figures. Or else what mattered was that I found friends close to home. Some were my age, others I formed into another female coterie of older women to be admired and adored. Then of course, I was just out of the hospital. Depressed, behind with my schoolwork, out of touch with my school friends, I'd found a new wave of

sympathy and interest. So, too, this religion gave me a struc-
ture of belief lacking at home. Moral imperatives became
my norms. Liberal provisos were wrong. Politics were irrel-
evant. Newspapers were missing the point. And the point
was (my stomach rolling around as I swallow and write the
words) — believe in Jesus Christ as Savior and Lord, or else
be damned.

My family found all this hard. I couldn't have chosen a
more effective form of teenage rebellion, the description
they used to console one another. I would brook no com-
promise with Mum, nor did I take kindly to teasing from
John. I was entrenched in absolutes they found repugnant
and none of us could find a graceful way around it. At first
there were frequent arguments. These petered out, to be replaced by an uneasy and unspoken agreement not to discuss
religion unless sorely provoked. It was too traumatic for all.
Mostly I still fought and played with Lucy and Jules as before. But there were times when I set out to convert them.
My little sisters were, by turns, bored and frightened when
I really turned on the heat, and were only spared more of all
this because of my discomfort with proselytizing. If somebody wanted to have the discussion, fine, but, however hard
I tried, I was uneasy and embarrassed when expected to declare the "truth" to an unwilling ear.

Sundays became centered on the church. Sometimes I
attended the morning service, always the evening one, and
the young persons' group afterward. Several evenings during
the week were given over to prayer and youth meetings, to
which I set off hot-foot on my bike, and later my motorbike.
I spent hours in my bedroom on my knees alone in prayer,

or listening to taped expositions of doctrine by the current Church favorites, or reading the Bible, or engrossed in badly written tales of evangelical courage, zeal, and piety. Distance lends enchantment, and the "saints" in these books performing their miraculous exploits were generally from the eighteenth or nineteenth century. I never thought I could match up to this crowd, but as more of the people I knew left to be missionaries, in Africa or Solihull, Afghanistan or Glasgow, I wondered whether that would be my lot too.

By the time I was sixteen, religion had become my sport. Come hell or high water, I was out there practicing it. I continued playing netball and tennis, but the floodlights had shifted. Then, during my first year of A-level exams, aged seventeen, studying hard and absolutely Christian, I lost my spine once again. This time it came out of the blue. One Saturday, away with my youth group, I sat in the lady chapel in Ely Cathedral overwhelmed by the presence of God. When evening came, once again I feigned an agonizing collapse. I slipped away from supper and immobilized myself on my camp bed. I was lying there in the hot hall, sweating and rigid, when they came to find me. The leaders were very worried, and after a sleepless night and a morning, I was taken by ambulance to the nearest hospital.

For a week or so I lay in a military hospital, alone and strangely exhilarated. I'd done what I had to do, now it was up to everyone else to sort it out. They could do nothing for me in Ely. Neither traction nor painkillers worked. I even crushed a water glass in my hand because of the "pain," and all these years later I can only guess what went through my mind doing this. Only for one moment was I frightened.

Two Christians I'd never met before (friends of a friend) prayed over me as I lay. Despite my great pain, unless I acted in faith, they said, God could never heal me. So I must get up and walk. I thought the man had seen through me. I did nothing and they left, with blessings.

My mother was away when this happened. She couldn't be contacted for days. John was beside himself with worry. He joked to me that as soon as my mother was out of the house, first the dishwasher broke down, then this. Somehow he visited me every day and finally managed to organize an ambulance transfer for me, to the London hospital I'd been treated in before. In the ambulance I played with two safety pins, fastening them through the top of my right hand. Once the skin succumbed to the point, it was a simple matter to ease the pin's shaft along beneath the skin's surface, then up into the air again, before closing it safely once more. When the nurses in London discovered these, they were horrified. I can still just make out the scars today.

The second operation happened much faster than the first. Another milogram was done; once again something showed up, or so I was told. Once again my back was cut open. Mum and John, anxious as hell, visited every day. My dad didn't show, of course. I was miserable. It was harder this time, recovering from the operation. Though I returned to school as fast as possible, for weeks I had to leave at lunchtime and take the bus back to the hospital for hydrotherapy. Now, finally, it came as a shock to me to find that my back really did hurt. I was frightened at last, frightened that I might have physically damaged myself with my own self-contempt. I never feigned back pain again.

Since then I have suffered backache, due, I suppose, to the damage caused by two unnecessary operations. Scar tissue lies beneath the double laddered lines climbing from the base of my spine. One day, if the pain gets bad enough for long enough, I'll take my courage in both hands and make a clean breast of it all. I suppose that's what happened to make me write this book. I don't relish being branded a fraud.

Those two operations must have been necessary to me. I don't know what I might have felt obliged to do otherwise. Maybe by giving all my attention to an imaginary physical pain, I could ignore a real one elsewhere, unnameable and untouchable. It was another kind of head-banging. And perhaps I hoped that if people were concerned enough about the agony in my back, somehow their concern would serve the other, unnoticed one. I was like a child playing a game of hide-and-seek. I made a good hiding place for myself by choosing a bad back. But it proved too good because no one ever found me out.

❖   ❖   ❖

This history seems like a series of notes from underground. On the surface I continued to perform the stable facts of my life quite cheerfully. After more or less recovering from the second operation I carried on with my studies. For a long while I found it hard to sit down at a desk for long periods and used to stand up during lessons. I even took my A-level exams standing up. Whether this was real or imagined physical discomfort, I can't now recall. I stayed on at school for a term after A-levels to take the Oxford University entrance exam. You could do that then, as long as you were at a private school. I was rejected by St John's College and nowhere else in Oxford would take me either. So I accepted an offer from another university, to study English. In the nine months I had free, I traveled to France, to ski, and to America, to see.

Replete with disappointment at my failure to get into Oxford, I began work before Christmas in a small, second-rate hotel in a first-rate French ski resort. I worked shifts as a receptionist and skied every day. At first all I could do with confidence in French was admire the view. This was no use for booking people rooms with shower, extra pillows, adjoining rooms, or extra towels. So the first weeks were alarming. The worst part was the telephone. My sign language didn't work here. As a disembodied voice, I couldn't try to look sweet, young, English, and incompetent. If somebody was organizing their skiing holiday, they weren't amused at being booked the wrong kind of room by a stuttering voice at the other end of the line. Once I'd mastered this small linguistic difficulty, however, I used the job to get what I wanted as ruthlessly as my boss used me.

If it hadn't been for my passionate affair with the mountains and the skiing (the closest in those days that I got to a passionate affair), I would have come home fast. I was racked by homesickness and wanted nothing more than to go home and live with Mum and John forever. Though I'd traveled between homes all my life, I felt painfully alone now. But I stayed for the three months, living in a broom closet behind the linen room on the second floor. When

March came I took the road down the mountain for the first time. I hadn't seen any earth or grass in that time. Snow had been over all. Catching sight of the first green field was like recovering one of my senses, though I didn't know it had been missing.

Soon after my return home, I took to the air again and spent my savings on America. For two months I toured on Greyhound buses, staying between friends. I fell in love with this country with all its array. On a brief trip beyond its borders, to Nassau in the Bahamas, I made my first, unwitting excursion into a terrain from which I sometimes feel I will never escape. I was staying with a family that was crisscrossed, like my own, by the lines of different marriages. But this family at this moment was fraught with fury. A stepfather and a stepdaughter (the same age as me) were locked in terrible combat. I was appalled by the things she would say about him, and by his contemptuous behavior toward her. These were performances my family had always fled from. Though I have never before connected this drama with the humble beginning of my own self-combat, the coincidence between the two now seems no coincidence.

One evening, after eating too much food, I found that I could simply regurgitate it back, down the toilet. I've got very strong stomach muscles and sometimes I've blamed them for the facility I discovered — that of being able, so simply, to rid myself of what I decided I did not want. The feelings of self-disgust that this performance produces were to come later. I had no idea that first evening that this small discovery would become the kind of compulsive nightmare I've lived with intermittently since then. It was as though I couldn't stomach what I was witness to. The feud between this unwillingly related father and daughter came too close to me and I had to try to separate myself from it.

Of course, my bulimic beginnings were partly to do with the passion for thinness that I, like everyone else in my world, suffer from. But the act of eating in order to relinquish what's been eaten, which began when I was nineteen, has to do with something else that is still with me now. Bulimia is a kind of double act, a compulsion that goes in two, apparently opposite, directions. First it's the urge toward, which is given in to, and then the equally violent urge against, which must also be conceded to. For a moment, eating too much appeases some hidden emotive void, as though I could consume the feeling itself. But the instant the eating has stopped, the food becomes unbearable to live with. Until I've rid myself of it, I feel ill at ease and bloated. The literal distension represents some terrible psychic distension. In being indescribable, this, I'm sure, comes close to the wordless horror at the heart of my breakdown after Jesse's birth.

This discovery made in Nassau has become another of my underground notes. Its furtive pattern has veered in and out of focus. Sometimes I have been free of it and sometimes not. It thrives on secrecy and is humiliated, even sent into brief exile, by candor. But the shame of such a confession makes it difficult to talk of a first time and even more difficult to admit to again. I don't understand why I have to do it, but by placing the fact of it alongside the other unappeasable parts of my story, perhaps I can dismantle its delusory appeal. Somewhere in the effort to describe I hope to make sense of events that seem opaque and disconnected from one another. Up until now, I have remembered my life as a series of rhetorics, each one discrete and with its own timbre. Writing them into one narrative I find myself listening for a common tune, albeit still a tune without words, somewhere underneath.

❖   ❖   ❖

During my first year at the university, I'd become uneasy with what I believed. I held the Christian fundamentalist line, but it was hard. I didn't want to get out, but I wanted my old certainty back. The rest of university life was comparatively straightforward. I liked my studies, friends, sports, and so on. Apart from the inevitable hiccups — an essay dropping in the university lake, a bit of sexual harassment, cash crises, somebody eating my food in the fridge — all was fine. It was just the religion that was such a difficulty. Christian friends talked of the "dark night of the soul" and "having one's faith purified by fire." They endeavored to reassure me and I clung on by my fingernails. Unfortunately I've inherited my fingernails from my mother — they are thin and splintery, not at all reliable when hanging over the abyss of unbelief.

In the summer term, I was baptized by total immersion. The setting was a large Nissen hut behind a handsome Georgian terrace. This housed my church. The water was warm, the hands that dropped me down and lifted me up felt strong. But as I stood beside my fellow swimmers, a line of earnest, happy faces dripping in white, an old man stood up from among the throng and addressed me: "I prophesy that your faith will be sorely tried in the next year and it will be hard for you not to be lured from the fold." For a moment I was sure he was a plant, put there by the pastor who knew some of my doubts. Then I chased the thought from my clean-sluiced mind and thanked God kindly for cautioning me.

I started my second year with a range of resolutions. One was to be less earnest in my studies, to let a little more air and pleasure in. Another was to write to my dad, whom I hadn't seen for an age. Feeling he'd given up on me, I wrote an angry letter. If he cared any more, I demanded he make contact with me. One morning in November I received a phone call from somebody I used to meet occasionally as a child and whom I hadn't seen for years. Tim was my stepmother's first husband and we encountered one another at those points of exchange that so often frame the life of the divorced child. I saw him when he returned my half-siblings (his children) to their mother (my stepmother) after they'd stayed with him. And sometimes, if it coincided with the end of my stay with my father, he gave me a lift home, back to my mother and stepfather in London.

When he phoned and asked to meet me that afternoon, I didn't think to ask why. I thought about it a little and assumed he must want to ask my student opinion about the city. Perhaps he was thinking of the city as a future site for his bookshop business.

The afternoon came. I cycled into the city center and met Tim, as arranged, outside a coffee shop. He was dressed somberly, in a dark suit and long overcoat. He didn't want to go in for a coffee and asked if we could go somewhere quiet to talk. I had no idea of, no apprehension about what he wanted to tell me. We found an almost empty lounge in a large hotel overlooking the cathedral. He began with the classic phrase, "I've got some very bad news to tell you," and still I hadn't an inkling. "Your father, Ivan, has been killed in an air accident in Saint Lucia." It had happened last Saturday, while I'd been playing a squash match, reading a book, laughing with my friends, and somewhere, at the back of it all, wondering whether Dad would answer my letter. I felt as though someone had knocked the wind out of me.

Dad had been in a small airplane with two other people, a father and son, on his way to a business meeting on another island in the West Indies. Though his great passion was flying and he was a good pilot, he was not the pilot for this last of all flights. The plane took off but never gained height. Tourists on the beach close by the airport had watched as the small plane crashed into the water close to shore. All three men were killed. They never discovered why it had happened.

I found it funny that I had to do all the things people do when someone close to them dies. Tim ordered a brandy, which I drank. I never normally drink brandy, and never at two in the afternoon. I needed, of course, to know all the details he had and kept asking questions I knew he couldn't answer, but which I had to ask. I hadn't seen Dad for about three years. I couldn't believe I could never alter that. His death was his ultimate unreliable act. I wept, and Tim consoled me as best he could. Two old ladies watched us. They couldn't have heard our conversation, but it was clear that a terrible drama was happening close to their tea-table and they were gripped. Their naked curiosity amused me. Even their tweed-suited, cucumber-sandwiched decorum couldn't hide it.

Mum and John were away when Dad died. So Tim, related to me by divorce, had traveled all that distance by train to tell me the news so I didn't have to hear it over the phone. After a couple of hours sitting in the pale green lounge, watching people look and look away as they realized that a piece of proper tragedy was happening in the corner, I pointed Tim toward the station. Then I unlocked my bike and cycled away. I cycled under a ladder. Nobody was up it. A workman called to me to watch out, it was bad luck to do that. I laughed at him through a blur of tears.

Tim had been relieved that I, like he, was a Christian. He thought, of course, that I would find consolation in my faith. But the death of my father also marked the death of God my Father. Without the one, I no longer needed the other, as though my father, alive, gave credence to God. Dad had had no kind of faith. Even somebody with liberal tenets would have been hard pressed to admit him to any community of believers. And I was no liberal. Yet I didn't believe he'd gone to hell. With my dead father standing up in the face of my belief, I no longer believed any of it.

My thoughts in the days after Dad's death have been washed away. I traveled to London and was looked after by my sixteen-year-old sister until my other parents returned home on the first available flight. My sister met me at the train, listened and talked to me and organized the meals. Though she never knew my father and found the whole business of my other family hard to comprehend, she responded to my trauma with extraordinary understanding, not of the thing it-self, but of her shocked and frightened sister.

When Mum and John returned, earlier in the morning than we'd expected, I was asleep in their bed. I hadn't wanted to sleep in my own room, up that extra flight of stairs. John was affronted to find me sleeping there and Mum had to mollify him, reminding him of the unusual circumstances. I went to Kent for the funeral. Tricia met me from the train in one of the vast, grumbling, crumbling diesel estate cars that still make me think of my father. I felt closer to her in the face of Dad's death than I ever had before, and that feeling has never gone. Our mutual jealousy had lost its object. In my stepmother's house, everybody was absorbed by their different grief. Though even now I felt my show of grief didn't match my brothers', I felt at home there. My brother Michael was just ten years old. He never spoke of his adored father the whole time.

Tricia had to identify Dad's body, flown back from Saint Lucia. She came back shaking. It hadn't looked like him. The face was bruised and swollen. There was to be an autopsy to establish the exact cause of death. It might have been a heart attack seconds before, or he might have died at the point of impact. She hoped it wasn't a heart attack, because he'd have hated to be thought of as a coward, someone who couldn't take the heat. He did die of injuries sustained on impact. But his death seems to me the only time he ever did take the heat. Most of his life was a different kind of flight.

I went to the funeral parlor and sat in a room with a goldfish tank, a Bible, a crucifix, some ugly gilt chairs, and my father's coffin. I wanted to open the lid and look inside but I didn't. I didn't know what I was meant to do there. It wasn't as though looking at this box would end anything. Dad's life had ended, but I'd be living with my memories of him till I died. He was to be cremated and the funeral took place in a huge, bleak, anonymous place. The vicar had never met Dad and it was clear that he'd failed to meet him imaginatively either. He conducted a superb pastiche of a service, quite as chilling as any satirical comedian could achieve. As the coffin descended, the machinery creaked. On one side of me stood my mother, dry-eyed. On the other, my grandmother wept loudly for the son who never forgave her, for what I never knew. In between, I wept, silently.

Afterward Grandma needed to show me her kid gloves with pink linings. They were beautiful and their soft leather cut a sharper place in Grandma's memory than her rough-edged, tormented, and unhappy son ever could. With the exception of her beloved husband Tommy, Grandma's life seemed shaped more by the cut and thrust of the tailor's scissors than by human intimacy. In the face of this, Dad's dogged scruffiness made sense. Maybe it was one of the best ways he knew to impinge upon his mother. Even so, I think he failed. I didn't go to see his ashes into the ground. I've never been to see where he remains. Right now I don't know who it would be I would be remembering.

Soon after the funeral, I returned to the university. My non-Christian friends were solicitous, but didn't know what to say. One of them cooked delicious food for me and hugged me wordlessly. My Christian friends had no words for me either. Their reassurances seemed specious in the face of the ruthless beliefs we all shared, but which I could not and would not now exercise. I didn't want to recover my belief and, over the next couple of months, put away even the last vestiges of religion. My loss of belief was exhilarating. Like Saint Paul locked up in jail, I found my chains suddenly cracked. Like him I climbed out of that gloomy, narrow place and into the light and the wind again. For a while I walked light-headed.

I'd met Hugh for the first time this term. He was my tutor for a course in eighteenth-century literature. I saw him the day I got back from the funeral, to talk about work I'd missed. He asked me if I'd like to go for a drink, maybe talk about my dad, if I wanted. He drank Irish whiskey to my shandy as I talked. He wasn't shocked by the black comedy of it all that drew hollow laughs from me. In keeping with that comedy, it's true that Hugh and I met over my dad's dead body. We saw each other again and again over the next few months and soon realized that our acquaintance was no longer casual.

Our love affair was furtive at the start, neither of us quite believing the other wanted to pursue it this far, and beyond. Few people knew about us as we traveled the countryside during those first months in Hugh's battered mini, seeking out places to talk and spaces to kiss all unobserved. I'd never imagined that my first adult love affair would be with a gay man, a man who for ten years had been coupled, Mr. and Mr., in the address on postcards he received. Now it had happened, his gayness was no problem. Before he'd fallen for Tom, Dick, and Harry, and now he'd fallen for me. I was much more worried by his cleverness than his sexuality. How will he keep on wanting me, I often wondered, when I can't talk as he can?

It took me a while to convince Hugh that he was no substitute for God or my father. He knew from the pictures that he didn't resemble either. But for me to lose both and come by him all within the space of a few months seemed too much of a coincidence. To compare Hugh to God, let alone my father, seemed so incongruous that it made me laugh out loud. And by way of showing him that he took the place of neither, and by way, for me, of surviving the death of each, we had many conversations about both. So it must be true that my grieving and my courtship walked hand in hand for a year or more.

I'd done much of this leaving and leavetaking just before I met Hugh. It took him longer to effect his. Yet despite the warnings that sang around my ears, that he'd never be able to make the break, however much he loved me, I never doubted he would. And he did, resolutely, stage by painful stage, till finally some two years after we met, we moved into our dusty and divided cottage.

Once my father was dead, I wanted to find out about him as I'd never thought to do when he was alive. Both my mother and stepmother, for their different reasons, began to talk as they never had before. And I found myself confronting a different man from the father I had known. On Boxing Day, one month after Dad died, I was on a walk through London with my family and some friends. I was unhappy and brooding, lagging behind in my own thoughts. Mum came up to me and told me to stop moping and put on a better performance for the occasion. I felt she was being a little abrasive, since Dad hadn't been dead very long. But I soon realized that her anger against him, though mainly dormant, was unabated. It seemed to me that she couldn't bear me to grieve over a man who had hurt her so badly. But he was my father.

As I heard more from these two mothers of mine, I was appalled by Dad's treatment of other women and amazed by the scale of his deception, inward and outward. Increasingly he seemed a sad, Walter Mitty figure, making up stories compulsively, often with little attention to plausibility. He'd paint himself as a single man with no children if he thought it suited, rather than the once-divorced married man with two children he actually was. He even bought the occasional engagement ring and went home to meet his betrothed's parents. Sometimes, it seems, he told lies where truth would have been easier. I still loved him, but I lost track of my own memories. I want to claim my father back again now, not as an idealized figure, but as someone who somehow loved me, despite the odds. I'd like to meet him posthumously and then be free to mourn him.

❖   ❖   ❖

When I decided to write a doctoral thesis, I chose for my subject a poet whose work I loved and about whom not much had been written. I didn't see then that I'd also chosen a figure who could embody my own preoccupations. Elizabeth Bishop died in 1979, so the closest I've ever come to meeting her is in my dreams. Nevertheless, in my thesis I've inscribed a woman whose life was shaped by her own unresolved childhood trauma. Though I didn't think of my own life in those terms when I wrote the thesis, something about her predicament, and the way she found to survive it, caught my attention.

Bishop wrote to defend herself from intolerable pain — the pain of surviving a childhood in which she felt "always a sort of guest." Her father died when she was a baby. Then her mother went mad. Her mother was committed to an asylum when Bishop was four years old and they never saw one another again. Despite her strong friendships and loves as a child and an adult, Bishop never left her terrible beginning behind her.

She asks the same questions again and again all through her writing. One of these is: Where's home? Now, looking back, I can see myself pondering the same question, seated at my desk in what was becoming the home of my own making, my first imagined and enacted home. I'd found myself settled, and in some ways happier, much earlier than I had expected to in the life I had invented with Hugh, as though I had answered for myself the question Bishop struggled with all her life. Though I wasn't free to travel in this life of mine, I was writing about someone who was always, of necessity and choice, a traveler, who for much of her life seemed profoundly displaced. My capacity to live a life so utterly different from that of my heroine left me with a strong ambivalence, as though I'd been robbed of the wandering that connected me with Bishop and that I was also so inwardly at home with.

Another question Bishop returns to is, what, if anything, lies beyond the visible fabric of the world? Hers is a tangible world whose frail, fragmented structures continually threaten to crumble and expose a hidden interior. It's as though she's always trying to keep at bay the chaos and dissolution she feels to be close at hand. It never occurred to me when I was writing my thesis that I'd ever describe my own life in those selfsame terms. Elizabeth Bishop recognized that her own terrible childhood formed her writer's eye. The poems she wrote rarely describe it, but her art is shaped out of it. As the hero of one of her greatest poems, "Crusoe in England," cries out, "Homemade, home-made! But aren't we all?" Now I wonder what I was so busy trying to defend myself against as I threw so much of my energy into making a home and then having a family, when so many of my contemporaries were busy escaping the same things. Whatever I was in flight from, it's nevertheless found its own voice and made its own space in my life. At first it seemed like a kind of terrible madness, but now it seems like a piece of myself.

Here is part of a poem Bishop wrote as an adult. It seems to express the extraordinary control she must have exercised, as a child, over her pain. This child displaces her grief; as though by placing it in a picture she can somehow manage it. The grandmother, so busy about the kitchen and her own grief, reminds me of how little the adults can sometimes bear to know. Sometimes, when I think of how much I still carry of all I felt as a child, I wonder what baggage my own small children are accumulating.

SESTINA

It was to be, *says the Marvel Stove.*
I know what I know, *says the almanac.*
With crayons the child draws a rigid house
and a winding pathway. Then the child

puts in a man with buttons like tears
and shows it proudly to the grandmother.

But secretly, while the grandmother
busies herself about the stove,
the little moons fall down like tears
from between the pages of the almanac
into the flower bed the child
has carefully placed in the front of the house.

Time to plant tears, *says the almanac.*
The grandmother sings to the marvelous stove
and the child draws another inscrutable house.

The child seems like an image for Bishop, who drew the outlines of different houses in her poems all her life as if to find an alternative to the one she'd known as a child. This child's house has a rigid inscrutability that is tied by the poem to a particular grief. Though it is alluded to in the grandmother's tears and the almanac's portents, it's unspoken of otherwise except in the child's sad pictures. Perhaps for Bishop writing poems was her only defense against going mad. If she could draw her own inscrutable houses, she would survive.

Alongside this subterranean loss she carried with her, Bishop also lived a life of pleasures and connections. Her letters, as well as her poems, are full of curiosity and passion. She teases and admires her friends, turning her sentences with wit and affection, and she celebrates her peculiar life, wherever it took her, with brilliant, hilarious idiosyncrasy.

The sadness I've talked about is like an underground note, resonating at a different frequency from the rest.

In my ambition to discover the roots of my breakdown, I've listened for one frequency while writing about my life and ignored the others. I'd never thought of it all like this before Jesse's birth. But then, I'd never thought of it all very much. In a way, looking back at my narrative, it's one neither I nor my family might recognize because my childhood was also a happy one with a clutch of good memories. But what I've done is a little like the milogram performed on me in the hospital. I've injected a dye down the backbone of my life and it's shown up a clutch of particular muscles, bones, and nerve endings. But it's left all the other parts and memories of my life invisible.

It's taken me the actual writing of this book to make me realize what I didn't realize when I started it — that all my life I have been displacing what I found impossible to bear. Why I should have broken down when other people, with worse lives, haven't, I don't know. Perhaps, finally, I was free to.

in search of
an illness

Never talk about it, don't read about it, if possible don't think about it." These were the injunctions given out to a friend of mine twenty years ago when she was discharged from the hospital unit treating her for anorexia. And for twenty years she adhered to them, more or less. As she pointed out, she must have needed to internalize them, feed on them maybe, or she wouldn't have listened so hard to her doctors' advice. I have taken the opposite course, equally necessary for my survival, and used my breakdown as the meat and drink of recovery. It is unthinkable to me to have done otherwise.

Before I became a psychiatric patient, I was skeptical about psychiatry. Electroconvulsive therapy sounded barbaric and nobody knew if it worked or how. Antidepressants might stave off unhappiness, but how could they touch the root of my misery? I understood that some people needed to be kept in the hospital against their will, but it never occurred to me that I'd be one of those people.

Once I was inside those psychiatric walls, my skepticism was like dust before the boulder of horror at the front of my mind. This was attacked with strong sedatives, high doses of antidepressants, and ECT. I was sectioned for a time, for my own safety. Though Hugh tells me that I continued to ask questions and tried to make sense of it all, nobody ever explained what they thought had happened or why they were treating me as they were. Curiosity was not a virtue. I was to accept it all as simply for my own good.

I never resisted the treatment. My cooperation wasn't necessarily expected, but it was given. I didn't want to treat myself well, as the bruises on my head testified, but I didn't stop others from legislating a "cure" for me. After all, after Christmas I went for ECT as a voluntary outpatient. There is a copy of the form with my shaky spider of a signature in unmistakable consent.

I was compliant and Hugh was compliant. It says so in my medical notes. It's not an adjective that I've ever heard used to describe either of us before or since. I never tried to avoid any of my sixteen ECT treatments, even though I was frightened each time. For someone as proud and independent as I am, it seems astonishing now that I allowed myself to be led to that horrible bed, to lie down and see people veering above me and knowing best, to suffer the pain in the arm and a moment of galvanized unconsciousness. And then wake to the pain in the head and not know where in my life I was. After these treatments, I was stunned and disoriented. After four and a half months of terrible depression and the dubious rigor of the cure, I seemed to Hugh like someone shell-shocked. ECT itself was its own kind of breakdown. My sense of identity had been so bombarded that it was impossible for me to have any continuous sense of myself at all. I couldn't piece my life together.

My anorexic friend's "pillar of salt" posture — on no account look back for fear of what your present might turn into — seems a strange one to me. One of my psychiatrists, Dr. B., wrote to my GP after I had requested psychotherapy: "This is really not my orientation and I [am] inclined to think that she should look ahead rather than back." But our present life is lived with the past in its heart. How could I make sense of what I was looking ahead at, when I was still so bewildered by what had happened?

Jesse was a year old when Dr. B. made this remark. For maybe a year after her birth I couldn't afford much curiosity beyond the dreaded confines of my mind. Though I hated the inside of my head, to allow my mind's eye to roam beyond it must have seemed too dangerous a liberty. Now, like Lot's wife, for the first time I was determined to look back.

When I was just out of the hospital, Jesse only two months old, I gave Hugh a jigsaw for Christmas, not the puzzle, but the saw. It was in conscious tribute to the little wooden table he had made for Eliza while I was in the psychiatric hospital. (What the unconscious attribution might have been, God knows.) But he had no time to cut shapes out of pieces of wood in the months afterward. His energy was taxed to its limits that spring as he made shapes for my life to help me live through it. Each day he worked to fill in the blanks, writing down who we would see and what we were going to do. So that even if I had no memory of having seen someone, or having been somewhere, it was written down and I knew it must have happened.

The following spring Jesse was a toddler, playing now with her sister at the little wooden table that stood, painted red, in the middle of the kitchen. Now I too sat down at my table upstairs and started to form my own jigsaw pieces, first turning over the jagged shapes and sounds from the months after Jesse's birth, then the more distant parts and fragments of my childhood.

While writing the first two chapters of this book, for as long as I was at my desk, I discovered a composure that was at odds not only with what I might be describing, but even with how I felt as soon as I stood up from my desk. In my sentences I could reclaim a piece of territory from the ravaged landscape of my mind. But in my life I still often felt myself to be a contemptible figure, unable to pretend to anything but her own blank unhappiness. Nevertheless it has been by way of words — my words — that I have gradually taken hold of my life. At my desk and in my psychotherapist's room, I've been forced to meet myself as never before.

I dreamed once that, while exploring a favorite cubbyhole cupboard in my grannie's house, I discovered a warren of attic rooms I never knew existed. They were full of things

I recognized and, quite at ease, I settled down to play. When I woke I was convinced the rooms were real. And even now, maybe ten years later, I am haunted by the sense that that house, as familiar to me as my own, has another story I've simply never found. Writing the first two chapters of this book, exploring back and back again, I have walked around my breakdown after Jesse's birth and my own life in rather the same way. I've discovered rooms, each connected to the last, that I'd never looked at before, and sitting at my desk, inhabiting them with words, I've found that they've changed the shape of the whole.

After six months of self-composition, I'd written all I wanted to for the time being, more than I thought I ever would about myself. I'd sat with my head sideways in my hands, gazing out of the window across the drystone wall of the garden, across to the ugly dull silver of our neighbor's barn, ransacking my head for the words that would express what had felt inexpressible after Jesse's birth. And, watching our neighbor come and go in his ancient jacket tied up with string, I'd made forays into the alarming territory of my own past, finding there the shapes of things to come. I still couldn't explain what had happened, but at least I saw that it had happened because I was me, living my life.

Now, and only now, did I dare lift the lid on psychiatry, as though what I had discovered and written down about myself gave me the confidence to look and see what the "experts" had come up with. Why had I been treated as I had? What did they think they were up to? And how on earth did any of it connect with what I knew of myself? By talking and writing I had started to inhabit my history, to possess it. But I was still the passive subject, still the patient, when it came to my psychiatric treatment, because I didn't understand it. Dr. A.'s refusal to see me and Dr. B.'s placebo answers only seemed to confirm this. I knew of only one way to get out from under this, and that was to master it. I decided to go out and research psychiatry and in particular to find out what had been said about my specialty, "postnatal illness." How did the psychiatrists understand my illness and its treatment? I'd check out bookshops and libraries, pick the brains of any friends or contacts I could think of who might be able to enlighten me more. I had no intention of writing a self-help book, but I thought I would be helping myself now if I could put myself in the picture.

The first thing I did was to look for books. I try never to have my children with me when I go into a bookshop. It drives us all mad. They can't share my interest, as they can for a short time if I'm buying food, clothes, or even curtain material. They know I've gone in beyond the covers, that I'm browsing territory they have, as yet, not even a toehold in. And when they try to seduce me back to them, telling me which covers they like the best, suggesting I buy some futuristic fantasy because it's got a dragon on the front, or something thick with letters embossed in textured silver, I've little patience. If I park them anxiously in the children's section for a moment, it's pandemonium. So when I entered the portals of Waterstone's in pursuit of psychiatry one hot Saturday in early June, I went in alone.

Ignoring my usual hunting ground, the tables and shelves of fiction, poetry, feminism, children, I sought a new set of spines. How very different one domain appears from another. I'd never walk up to the Computing shelves, mistaking them for Art History. I can usually spot Gender Studies at a hundred paces, though just occasionally I might find myself in Sociology by mistake. Poetry is impossible to mistake, all those thin stripes of color. Psychiatry, though, I had to rummage for. I'd never browsed in this before. When I found it, dispersed here and there, among "Psychology" (chance would be a fine thing), it seemed to have no anxiety about itself. Apart from Anthony Clare's *Psychiatry in Dissent,* which I also bought, the titles declared no doubts. There were at least half a dozen introductory textbooks with titles like *Essential Psychiatry, A Handbook for Trainee Psychiatrists,* and *Problem Based Psychiatry* (how psychiatry can solve them). I chose two from the shelf: Gelder, Gath, and Mayou's *Concise Oxford Textbook of Psychiatry* and Jennifer Hughes's *Outline of Modern Psychiatry.* Then I came home in great excitement, thinking that maybe now I'd be able to make sense of my treatment.

Sitting in the garden that same day, I began to read. At first I was amused by the academic and reductive accounts of human behavior. I read bits aloud, somewhat incredulously, to Hugh and some friends in the garden. Then, despite the sun, despite the laughter, I was chilled.

There was no skepticism and no psychology. Lives, it seems, can be described as illnesses and organized in just the same way as organic diseases would be. If these lives are sufficiently unhappy or out of order, then they become a series of symptoms, classified, placed within an etiology, named as a disorder, and treated, in my case with psychopharmacology (sedatives and antidepressants) and ECT.

To find out about my own "illness," I turned to the chapter in the *Outline of Modern Psychiatry* called "Disorders of Female Reproductive Life." There, in the space of a page, I found myself categorized: definition, frequency, predisposing factors, causes, clinical features, treatment, and prognosis, all given relatively clearly, for "puerperal psychosis." I understand the psychiatrists' dilemma — they have to find a way of organizing the range of mental trauma and crisis that comes their way. Nevertheless it was dismaying to find my experience boxed in like this, reduced to an implausible scientific jargon. As though by imposing their "scientific" language on someone, they could make sense of and contain all the fever and the fret. I read both books from cover to cover, though I soon stopped reading bits out loud. But far from having conquered anything, I was mystified. They offered me no explanations, either for my "illness," or for my treatment. Psychiatric practice seemed more like an exercise in damage control than an effort to find a cure.

But what my reading did do for me was to make the shift I'd been looking for. Now I was no longer a patient, in the grip of psychiatry. Now I was a person and determined to understand what had happened, even in the face of my own precarious self-respect and horrible memory loss, despite the ignorant renditions of psychiatry.

Soon after my psychiatric garden party, a bulky brown envelope came in the mail containing the medical records compiled during the two months I had been in the hospital after Jesse's birth. I'd written to the Patient Services Manager asking for copies of them, explaining that I was writing a book and needed to counter the gaps in my memory due to ECT, depression and all. I thought the notes could fill in some of my blanks and I was most curious to know what had been said about me.

The notes arrived quite promptly, but if I'd thought I might find myself in them, I was disappointed. What I found was a case, scrupulously documented, impressively detailed. The person I'd searched for in my memories of the hospital was not there. If the nurses had borne witness to what I was going through, and some of them did, in the notes they had translated me into a mental patient with objectively ascertainable symptoms. I displayed "inappropriate behavior," sometimes making "good eye contact" or "over-intellectualizing illness but [with] obvious deficient logic when discussing her eating." At other times I was "quite vacant" or "tearful," "hostile-looking" or "uncommunicative." I was often "very low" or, as the doctor would put it, had a "depressed affect." As I "improved," I started holding "appropriate conversations," being "patient" with Jesse, and my "mood" became "bright" or "brighter." My relationship to Jesse was described mainly in terms of my practical engagement. I "fed," "bathed," and "cared" for her. My thoughts and feelings about my predicament were sometimes recorded, but not because they had any status in determining the problem. Only as part of the "mood" record.

But I wasn't content with just reading what the doctors had to say about my depression. What about other women who'd been through something comparable to me? What had they found to say about their predicament? Maybe I'd understand my own experience differently in the context of other women's lives. So during the summer and into the autumn, alongside my psychiatric research, I contacted other women I had come across, directly and indirectly. I even thought that perhaps I could include their accounts with my own.

Only one woman was unwilling to meet me, so we talked for a short while on the phone. She'd been in the psychiatric unit two years before me, "mad as a hatter" after the birth of her daughter. Her female GP had told her to be grateful for what she'd got and never to have a second child. But now at last she had dared to get pregnant again and changed doctors. She didn't want to talk about what had happened the first time because it always made her feel worse and she wanted to do all she could to forget it. But she recalled her terror of two things in particular while she was hospitalized: the ward round, when people talked about her as though she was on show; and ECT — when she was electrocuted and left alone, with no help and no explanation.

The other women, from new mothers to grandmothers, talked to me in all kinds of places: in my home at Fisher's Yard, in the Blacksmith's Arms, over a pizza in the Pizza Express, walking along a beach on a bright, cold afternoon, and once in a small, hot, and oppressively clean house less than half a mile from the highway overpass that had nearly been the death of my companion. She told her story against the clock, trying to give it all before her husband came back, and in the face of her own bewilderment. Even though she'd nearly killed herself and spent months in psychiatric and general hospitals as they stitched up her body, shocked her, and drugged her mind, even though she'd been told she'd now be on lithium (a powerful mood-stabilizing drug) for life, nobody had taken the time to tell her what they thought had gone on. Or asked her much about her thoughts and feelings. An Austrian woman who'd moved to England to be with her English partner, she felt herself to be not only a stranger in a foreign land, but now a stranger to herself.

It was an odd experience, listening to strangers recalling something they'd rarely talked of to anybody else. I saw them wrestle, as I had done, with an experience that they found impossible to connect with their love for their child and hard to make any sense of. Nevertheless, what they had to say confirmed my sense that while "postpartum depression" often arrives as though a bolt from the blue, it rises out of the fabric of each of our lives. And it's more deeply inscribed in the fabric of social life in our culture than is ever remotely acknowledged.

When in the depths, I saw myself as a strange and solitary being performing a terrible, ungainly dance. Wrapped up in a black cloak, I thought I was the only star in this particular dark sky. As I've recovered myself and shrugged my shoulders out of that awful introversion, I've noticed how dense a constellation of other women is clustered around me. I seem to have been inducted into a silent community. There are so many others, both at first and second hand, who have suffered some form of deep misery after the birth of a child, more than I would possibly have imagined. Some have lived with their unhappiness, telling nobody except perhaps their partner or doctor, and come out the other side; some were put on medication but managed to stay at home; some, like me, had to be hospitalized and so have additional traumas to recover from, like ECT or the stigma they experience of having been in a mental hospital; and the occasional person I have been told of did not survive to tell any tale.

Almost all the women I've talked to say they don't understand what has happened to them. Those that have asked can't get anyone to explain it to them. Many still find their lives jarred by the strange and terrible mood that began with the birth of their baby. They are no longer incapacitated by it, but it wasn't there before the birth and it hasn't gone away since. During the worst time, most, if they can, lock away their misery, exhaustion, bewilderment, and fear behind a carapace that manages to function, if only just. Some are still wondering, over a decade later, whether they will ever recover from whatever it was that happened after that day still so often described as the best in a woman's life. Perhaps I was lucky that even the carapace gave way.

Though many of the accounts were as stark and dramatic as any storyteller could have wished, I couldn't use them directly. Each time it was quickly apparent that what someone was telling me about was not some strange interloper of an illness, arriving in the middle of their life from nowhere. Their depression was the expression of something unbearable in the midst of it all, letting rip. The manifest features of each woman's breakdown were nothing beside the frustration, loneliness, and misery most felt at being tongue-tied and ignored. So, though I have not described anybody else's history, these other stories have consolidated my belief that the black flower of "postpartum depression" has its roots thrust deep into the soil of each person's life.

That same summer I spoke to an eminent geneticist. He was a distant but familiar neighbor during my growing-up years. He had children about my own age. For years before running was fashionable, he and his wife used to flash slowly past our house as they jogged their requisite distance each day. They never changed their clothes. He was still dressed in shirt, trousers, and lace-up shoes and she in skirt and blouse. I'm not sure whether she even changed her shoes, though her low-heeled summer sandals would surely have been too dangerous. Eventually they capitulated to matching sweatsuits and running shoes, but only after I had left home.

Mum had talked to this geneticist neighbor during the first months after Jesse's birth and he had assured her that I was genetically predisposed to my "illness." This was because my maternal grandfather was depressive and because Mum had had one depressive episode when I was about twelve. I was interested to know how he explained this dismayingly deterministic model and by now I felt equipped to deal with such an encounter. So I arranged to talk with him when I was next down in London. We finally had our chat during the wake-party my mother and stepfather had organized to try to celebrate our leavetaking of our beloved family home.

He didn't take me very seriously, not nearly as seriously as I took myself. He saw our brief exchange more as a form of soft flirtation. He asked me what I was up to, and I told him what I had been writing and why I wanted to talk to him. I wanted to know what he, as a chemical pathologist interested in genetic predisposition, had to say about what I had experienced. And I wanted some suggestions for further reading.

This emeritus professor told me that what I had been writing was very worthwhile if it made me feel better, but of no basic use in understanding why I had suffered a breakdown. It might be a placebo, but nothing more. I had a genetic predisposition to depression, and childbirth just happened to be the trigger. He seemed to think that any other traumatic event would have done just as well. As far as he was concerned, neither pharmacology nor psychotherapy were of much use, because you get better from depression in the end anyway. He expressed himself in a tone of exquisite, unconscious condescension. There was no question that his might not be the only story, so he could be generous to those like me whose notions were so fetchingly far-fetched.

Our conversation was, inevitably, short because of my ignorance about his expertise and because he didn't seem very engaged by my project. But he did direct me toward the books that might enlighten my psychiatric ignorance of the "illness" I had labored under. And he gave me the names of various people I might talk to, advising me to use his name freely as recommendation. So when I returned to my study, I started ordering books and articles and writing letters to different people and organizations. This was something I knew how to do. I'd spent years of my life filling in library forms and skimming piles of books, looking for the nuggets I needed. I was at home here and in control.

Some of the books and articles I ordered never arrived. But after several months immersed in those that did, I felt I'd had enough. I understood, theoretically, what kind of beliefs underpinned psychiatric practice in England. And I read enough to be able to chart for myself the shape of psychiatric debate about motherhood and mental illness. Some of the papers had left me a little cold, such as "Epidemiological Aspects of Mental Illness Associated with Childbearing." But I read through them nevertheless. Even a paper by our neighbor on "Endocrine and Bio-chemical Studies in Puerperal Mental Disorders," which meant little to me at first, took its place in my field of knowledge. Admittedly, having read it through, I arranged to go to the pub with a biologist to be sure I understood the implications of what my neighbor and his co-author were saying.

A few names came up again and again in my reading and it became clear that a handful of psychiatrists in England and abroad are responsible for an extraordinary amount of the academic and practical research that has been done into the condition of "postnatal illness" in recent years.

My decision to read and write about psychiatry was partly a wish to cover my back. By this time, I was hoping that what I had written would one day become a book. I didn't want anybody to be able to accuse me of not having looked at the psychiatric evidence. But all this reading also formed part of my internal journey. I was no longer the unwitting object of somebody else's expertise. I understood my psychiatrists' terms, and I was able now to stand back and form my own, if retrospective, opinion about them.

Though I've met several psychiatrists for whom I have a great deal of respect, I am not a convert. Psychiatry's dogmatic adherence to a language of science and its search for facts still seems bizarre to me in the face of the lives it attempts to categorize. As though working in the opposite direction to psychotherapy, psychiatry tries to make each individual fit into a medical generality. Once a person's behavior has been given the appropriate technical term, they can be forgotten about as someone with a particular life and treated as a condition instead. This is understandable given the scale of medical demand and the drastic under-resourcing of the National Health Service, but it still leaves the patient in the lurch.

In the thick of all my reading I felt sometimes as though I were joining in a child's game. Eliza plays elaborate charades for hours, during which she invents fantastical landscapes using whatever comes to hand. To play with her you have to suspend your sense of what things are usually used for and how they fit into the ordinary world. I've never tried to play the psychiatric game as much as I have played Eliza's. But that game, like hers, seems intent on describing things in its own exclusive language. Either you play with it, or it seems utterly mystifying. But the key difference between Eliza and the psychiatrists is that she depends on fluid shifts of parameters and a constant reimagining of her objects. And she doesn't think that a child who doesn't want to play her game is wrong for wanting to play another.

Once I started writing, I soon discovered how difficult it was to represent psychiatric ideas without seeming complicit in them. At first I was sucked into the very language I wanted to provide a critique of. I drafted and redrafted the chapter as I tried to establish in my writing the distance from psychiatry I felt in my mind. The effort to give clear expression to this material became a hiatus. Just as psychiatry seems to have little to do with my recovered sense of myself and to have offered me nothing by way of understanding what went on, so the writing about psychiatry seemed out of place in my story. So having written a chapter of it, packed with footnotes and quotations, I moved it. First I moved it from the middle of the book to the end, then into an appendix, and finally I took it out altogether. Though I can't be rid of my memory, or lack of memory, of psychiatric treatment, and though I will never know how much my survival was due to that cocktail, I can at least displace psychiatry in my narrative and leave my own language intact.

I was in London the following November to celebrate my mother's graduation, a month after Jesse's second birthday and only thirty-five years later than Mum would have wished. So I arranged meetings with two of the people whose names I had come across during my research. Clare Delpech set up and runs a charity called the Association for Post-Natal Illness that offers support and advice to women in any kind of state after childbirth. Channi Kumar heads the Mother and Baby Unit at the Maudsley Hospital and is vitally involved in the research being done into postnatal illness. Both are well known for their work with women suffering from postpartum depression. If I talked to them, I thought, surely I could cover the inadequacies I was sure must be rife in the psychiatric profile I was assembling.

Leaving my children for the day in London was a novel experience. I dressed and packed my bag as though embarking on a piece of investigative journalism, so disguising one project to myself inside the uniform of another. Maybe I thought I'd gain some new insight from these two expert witnesses. That's certainly what I told myself. But much more important was my determination to situate my psychiatric treatment. Perhaps I also thought that these two interviews would give me material for a form of writing I can't do. Somehow I'd find a language of altruism and self-help that I know now I don't possess.

I set off for the subway with my heart beating high in my chest. I had notebooks, pencils, cash, mints, a street map, and, most important, an unwieldy borrowed tape recorder. I looked the part to myself. Glancing back, I might have cut a comic figure. But at least it was me who was doing the investigating now. Beneath my V. I. Warshawski parody was a woman determined to take on and understand the "illness" that had incapacitated her. A year earlier I'd never have believed I could make the journey I made that day, on my own terms and in my own way.

By the time I reached Parsons Green, I was sweating. With a little time to kill, I wandered up and down relentlessly residential streets close to my first appointment. I was searching for somewhere to browse the minutes away. My bag was heavy with journalistic fantasies and I dropped it in a shop selling smart second-hand children's clothes. For maybe ten minutes I pretended to be a mother with different children, the kind that wear tulle for parties. I didn't let on that I was from out of town, but I think the shop assistant had my number. I couldn't rub the dung from my boots that easily. By the time I left, I knew I could no more drop my self and pretend to a different kind of interest, whether in party frocks or postpartum depression, than I could fly.

I went to the wrong house first. The right number in the wrong street. An immensely tall woman with stiff and expensive blonde hair answered the door. Behind her a man in overalls was about to topple beneath the large cardboard box he was carrying up the stairs, and other boxes were waiting. She wasn't pleased to be mistaken for somebody else who ran an organization for postpartum depression. It was not a good beginning for my would-be detective self.

The front room of Clare Delpech's home is cluttered with all the paraphernalia of what seems, to a stranger, to be a life spent on the run. Books, records, and pieces of paper, a piano with music heaped, tables and bookshelves piled with files, boxes on the floor equally full, an open, packed filing cabinet, a word processor, family photographs, cold cups of tea, the occasional piece of decorative china that didn't get out when the going was good, a tennis racket, stereo system, newspapers, and a shabby, comfortable three-piece suite. She has five children, all still at home, her own printing shop to manage, a doctoral thesis to research in biochemistry, and a charity to head. After the birth of her third child, in 1979, she became, in her own words, hopelessly suicidal. She survived this, but could find out nothing about her diagnosed condition. So to confront this "conspiracy of silence, not least from women themselves," she set up the charity, even as she had her fourth and fifth children and corresponding bouts of depression.

Clare talked for a couple of hours, with my tape recorder making a quiet, ratchety noise on the floor. I learned a little

about her and something about the charity, but nothing I
didn't already know about the "illness." At least that confirmed that my research so far had covered the right ground.
I left the house relieved that I had no wish to be worthy. It
demands so much repetition. The conversation I had with
Clare is one she must have had thousands of times. Yet her
gusto suggests she hasn't tired of it yet. As for me, it confirmed what I knew underneath: that I am not writing my
book out of charity.

Whenever I am nervous, my stomach turns to water. I
made the journey to Denmark Hill, home of the Maudsley
Hospital, by way of several inconvenient conveniences,
"public convenience" being the term used by the British
authorities, for reasons that seem obscure, for public toilets.
I had compiled a list of questions to raise with Professor
Kumar and as I sat on the crowded bus from the Elephant
and Castle, my bags heaped on my knees, I went through
them. I had to hold my papers almost to my nose because
the man sitting beside me had his elbow stuck into the space
above my lap as he read his paper.

Having found the Institute of Psychiatry, I climbed its
steps a few minutes early. My name was phoned up by a surly
porter and I sought out the last in my line of "conveniences."
Then I sat in the foyer, which reminded me of my university
days, with signs to lecture halls, leaflets about courses and films
lying about, and students, or "new grown-ups" as Eliza calls
them, crisscrossing my line of vision. But unlike the universi-
ties I'd studied at, here I'd have been the subject of study. I sat
waiting for Professor Kumar to come and find me and
thought how purposeful these adolescent psychiatrists

looked, with their briefcases and files. Then I wondered how they saw me. "They must think I'm a patient," I thought, "I'm not dressed in formal clothes, they must think I'm a psychiatric case. So I got out my notes and mimicked the scholarly attention that would surely convince anyone glancing my way that I sat on their side of the fence. This from someone who thought she didn't believe in the fence. And had been on the other side of it.

When Channi Kumar arrived, he shook my hand gently and firmly. He was courteous, softly spoken, and dressed in clothes that had a reassuringly scruffy edge: worn and baggy brown corduroys, shirt, tie, and sweater. We traveled the corridors to reach his office, a small room only a little larger than my own study. It was lined with books and files and dominated by a large, ungainly wooden desk on the right, one of those desks with secret drawers. He asked me why I wanted to see him and I explained a little of my project and how I had come by his name. I asked him whether I could use my tape recorder. He didn't refuse permission, but made it clear he would prefer me not to. So after a little toing and froing, looking for electric sockets and fiddling with wires, I put it away. He suggested I take notes instead. A sure sign I am not cut out for journalism is my incapacity to take notes. I've never been able to lift out the salient details, whether from a book, lecture, or conversation and this meeting was no different. I opened my notepad, but when I closed it an hour later, nothing was written down there.

This eminent psychiatrist, known worldwide as an authority on postpartum depression, whose articulate mission I had been so impressed by in my reading, whose name cropped up everywhere, listened to my questions very carefully and replied without condescension. He, in turn, asked his own. The details of my psychiatric history, features of my depression, how soon it had happened, how I had been treated, how long I had taken antidepressants, who my psychiatrist was. He didn't seem particularly interested in what I was writing or how. More that the fact of me doing it symbolized a degree of recovery. He asked me whether I had my medical notes. He was careful not to poach on somebody else's patch, by seeming to advise on another doctor's case, but couldn't see why there should be a problem with publishing them.

When he thought I was criticizing my treatment, he began to reprimand me a little. I should be grateful that I lived in England and had gone into the hospital *with* my baby. I reassured him that I was. He affirmed the use of ECT for women like me. But alongside ECT, treatment of inpatients in his unit also always included some kind of psychotherapy or counseling, often for the father as well as the mother. A far cry from my experience. He acknowledged that the line between severe "postpartum depression" and "puerperal psychosis" could be very fine. And though he used to think he could always identify a psychosis, now he wasn't so sure. Though Professor Kumar seemed immensely confident and authoritative, it was something new to me to hear a medical doctor speak, if only for a moment, of his own uncertainty. I left his room knowing he was someone to be respected and I was impressed that he had treated me similarly.

While we talked, a child screamed, again and again, a long, drawn out note. Channi Kumar gave no sign of having heard. Maybe it was something familiar in that place. It cut through me, this scream not of a tiny child, but of someone maybe seven or eight years old. I couldn't tell whether it was a girl or a boy. Its cadence didn't change and sounded the more terrifying for its lack of urgency. It was like a cry that had to be voiced but which didn't expect to be heard.

I wrote my notes on the bus back to Elephant and Castle in jerky lines. Even when the bus was stationary, my hand shook. Professor Kumar had been courteous, helpful, and generous to the last. My meeting with him had been as good as I could have hoped for. But the child's cry stayed in my ears like a shape I didn't know the name of. I'm sure I never screamed out loud like that as a child. Only as an adult. But the screaming I did in other shades when I was small was never heard. The child's noise rang through my body, like the echo of something I had never been that far from and that I had come all too close to since Jesse's birth, first in my break-down and then in my writing.

It seems paradoxical to say that my writing has been, in some way, close to a scream. Not that it is one, but that it's been trying to make sense of what it was that took me be-yond words. Yet it's a preoccupation that's been with me for so long. Two years after my father died, I wrote an essay about Herman Melville called "The Scream." It seemed to me then that for some of Melville's figures, like Pierre, Bartelby, and Billy Budd, the possibilities of language even-tually gave out, and they were forced beyond language into a scream of action. Like Münch's figure in his picture *The Scream,* they ended up, paradoxically, forever screaming in terror and forever silent.

At the time it didn't occur to me that I might be writing as much about myself as about Melville's characters. About some trauma submerged within me that had gone beyond language, beyond my capacity to make sense. Even when I went on to write about Elizabeth Bishop and to place a scream she puts at the heart of her story "In the Village" at the heart of my doctoral thesis, even then I thought I was writing only about my beloved poet. But in the end, sitting in the psychiatrist's office and hearing the invisible child, the scream that stayed in my bones was mine, not theirs.

Reaching Elephant and Castle I traveled along the black and red of the subway lines to Notting Hill Gate. I was on my way to meet Adam for the evening. It was seven o'clock and I walked the long, straight pavement with its shuttered antique shops in a mood of euphoric exhaustion. While I was still only pin-size in view, a man appeared, running toward me. Then behind him, a woman, also running. He was running a little faster than she. As he came closer, I could hear her shouting, "Stop him, stop him, thief, thief. He's taken my bag, help help." Again and again she cried out. By now he was within twenty meters and I had to consider what to do. It was clear that the man had the woman's bag. There it was, a bulge tucked into his open jacket, only partly concealed.

I did nothing. I even stopped walking, and I watched first the man, then the woman, run past. As he jogged past, self-contained, silent, and with little apparent sense of urgency, we exchanged glances. His was as knowing as mine. He took me in his stride. When she ran by, everything was out. She was untucked, her arms flailed, and her voice sounded far away in the thin November air. She saw me only for the moment it took her to go by. Her brow was raised and mouth agape at this treacherous familiar place that was turning its back on her violation, her loss.

Two minutes later I arrived at Adam's apartment. Everything seemed normal. The Serene Fish Bar and Nahal's were open, as usual. Adam was in a chair beside the window two floors up, a book in his hand, as usual. I rang the bell. Then, sitting on the floor amid a clutter of books, with a glass of wine, I told Adam about my day. I joked that it always paid to have a psychoanalyst, like him, on hand when going to see a psychiatrist. And I said that I was disconcerted, because I thought I'd been researching one thing — my own illness — only to find that, like a palimpsest gone awry, the layers of my life kept breaking through.

❖   ❖   ❖

The psychiatrists were never interested in the words I chose. Words had only one side to them, as far as they were concerned; storymaking was all very well so long as it didn't go too far. It was, perhaps, advisable not to make a habit of it. So they found out very little about me, and so did I.

When I started talking to Anna, my psychotherapist, fifteen months after Jesse was born, the words I used about myself began to take different shapes. Sometimes they were shapes I agreed with, but often not. I found myself saying things I wanted back, inside me. The thoughts and feelings I tried to give voice to wouldn't sit still. And when I felt utterly distraught, it was still nearly impossible to give a voice to my feelings at all. Sometimes this left me weeping, or so tight — with anger or loneliness — that I clenched myself. Then often I'd change the subject. Suddenly my attention would be caught by a crack in the ceiling, or the shadow thrown in a picture, or the slant of a plant beside the watery bowl of shells. Neither of us was fooled by this shift. But I know now how much my spirit takes refuge in the material landscape. I cling on, with my eyes if not my hands, to the grain of what I can see.

I was always more likely to turn up early than late, so I had my own rituals for killing that extra time. Sometimes I went to buy groceries near by, enjoying the unaccustomed liberty of doing it by myself. It's so much easier to browse the vegetables, brooding about fennel and petite turnips, without attendant children. I could sample with my eyes the different kinds of tahini or salami I might buy when I didn't have a child trying for a different kind of sampling. If my time was too short for this kind of luxury, I parked the car a little distance from Anna's house and got out a book. For a while I often wrote a list of things I wanted to say because the frustration of forgetting them once inside that room was more than I could bear. But however I filled the minutes before my session, my stomach still turned upon me when I pressed the bell.

For months and months I took myself, always very promptly, to Anna's front door twice a week, rang the doorbell, and went into her front room, there to take my place on a sofa and experience terrible devastation. And after fifty minutes I had to get up and go. I left my therapist in every kind of mood, but I always left.

Anna's house was one in a long terrace of white-gray brick leading uphill. It had a small front garden packed untidily with shrubs and flowers and a tall pine tree in the far corner. Sometimes there was an empty potato chip bag or crushed can in among it all. In the neighboring house I often saw a young woman ironing clothes in the front room and a small child, and I wondered whether the hourly doorbell next door got to her through the week. What she made of all these people paying visits to her neighbor.

The room was always the same. That's not quite true, because the plants grew and sometimes there were more cat hairs on the low table in the middle of the room. The water was renewed in the bowl of shells to the right of the fireplace. And once a month there was a small square of paper for me, a bill, positioned parallel to one edge of the table. The floor was stripped pine and rugs. This front room was divided from another by big wooden doors, securely fastened. In one corner stood a single speaker, a plant decently obscuring much of it from my view, silent witness to a life beyond the consulting room. In the other room, the back room, which I never saw, stood its partner. And when I was not there, there was space for different sounds to be made.

After starting my twice-weekly pilgrimage to the hunting ground, or shrine, of my hidden self, I didn't discover any new facts about my life, or "life-events," as my psychiatrists would describe them. What I did discover is how much I construct the life I live around my capacity to tolerate the root pains that trouble me. When I was a teenager, I took refuge in a form of agony I could identify and gain respect for, and laid myself low with my "very bad back." And after Jesse was born the pains once again became unbearable. Unlike the antidepressants, the psychotherapy didn't dull the pain. Instead it's made it harder for me to avoid my own distress.

I was often taken aback by how banal some exchange between the two of us might seem, yet leave me choking on a phlegm of anger or on the hard pip of loneliness. And those now familiar furies struck as easily out of a sunny day as out of a storm. However, when my fury and sense of bereavement seemed legitimate, I didn't find myself so much at their mercy. One important insight I drew from this expensive conversation was that if I could listen to the sound of my rage, even though I didn't like what I heard, maybe I could affirm it. Like the smell of my own shit, it was a necessary, even enjoyable, product of the person I am.

I still have a superstitious worry that to affirm a pleasure too strongly will result in some unpleasant reprisal. I'll get the runs. But if I can suspend that superstition for the duration of this sentence, I will say that my time every week in that same front room has made a positive difference to my life. It's hard to say quite how, especially as for so long what I experienced on that sofa was so hard to take. As was I.

I don't think I knew what my past was composed of before I started the twice-weekly visits. I didn't dare look at much of it. Although I knew that the breakdown after Jesse's birth must, like Jesse, have been born out of me, I couldn't make out how. Or why that birth at that time should have been too much to live with. Though I had plenty of worries about being the mother of two children under two, without a job or an income, a city girl living in a small village far from my family and closest friends, it never occurred to me I'd not be strong enough to manage.

It's no coincidence that shortly after I began the psychotherapy, I also began to write. Those two spaces each week licensed my writer's curiosity about myself, never till then given air. What began as an article, describing my memories of the weeks after Jesse's birth, rapidly grew beyond this first design. At each stage, when I have talked of my fear of writing more, fear of what I might say, Hugh, or Hermione, or Adam has said, "Just write it. You can always put it away, never show it to anyone." But I think they knew as well as I that by writing it, I was taking it beyond that private place that no one sees.

So this talking and this writing have occupied parallel tracks. My speech in Anna's front room has been shaped by ebbs and flows, interruptions and contradictions, circling and uncertainty. By contusions of grammar and experimental rambles that trail off into unfinished silence. Things get said again and again, banalities are rife, and it matters not a whit. Even my own boredom has its place. The process of writing is very similar. But in the end, I leave certain words on the page, in a certain order, and they are fixed. Their meaning is not fixed but they are. And unlike the sentences I speak and lose, the ones I invent on the page are there to stay. Here more than anywhere else, I feel able to fight free and speak of myself as I discover I wish to. With this act of composition I can craft my own composure, one I feel at home in. That has been the source of my excitement in writing this book.

I have always been a keeper of deadlines. But when I started writing my own lifeline I failed my first one. Hermione had helped me secure my "madwoman" project, the *Jane Eyre* edition, and I'd worked on it for four months or so in my available piecemeal time. Though I never got close to completing it, this task, complete with contract, gave me an important reminder. Though my life still seemed confined by a horizon that extended no further than my own literal and metaphorical threshold, it needn't always be bounded so.

However, once I started inventing my own story, *Jane Eyre* was placed on the shelf. I was shocked that I'd put it so far from my mind when Hermione reminded me of it, four months from the deadline, and suggested I ought to decide whether to complete it or not. To do so would have meant abandoning my other writing and my decision was made. I could no more leave what I was doing than leave myself. So I had to pass Jane on to someone else, better able to listen to and write about her sighs and exclamations, and carry on pursuing my own. The ease with which I failed one commitment served to confirm the other.

❖   ❖   ❖

As I started to write, I began to search for company. I needed it. I became aware of a world in which other people had done similar things and other writers had found their own narrative ways of owning and owning up to their experiences. How had they given voice to a trauma that sometimes seems to me to be an unspeakable predicament and often to defy articulation? How had they managed their own falling apart? Although the tales I came across were a far cry from my own, still I needed to shape companions in my mind.

My interest then was still tentative and even now I can find it as disturbing to walk the corridors of someone else's madness as I do to return to the corridors in which some of my own madness was lived. A newspaper article just as much as a book-length autobiography can leave me uncertain of my own hold. I still find myself seduced by the echo of my own breakdown, as though it had some tidal pull on my mind. So my curiosity, set in motion by my own search for the sentences, has been bounded by the shifting limits of my own toleration.

The return of my memory helped shape my reading. I began to dare a little more when the book I had read at night still had some place in my head the following morning. It was as though I'd recovered some lost tongue. I used to make a joke of it with Hugh and with friends, that if they — or I — wanted to know what I thought of a book, they'd have to speak to me before it was cold from my hands. But, like the best jokes, it was also deadly serious and there were times when I wondered whether I'd ever again be able to read as I had done. Sometimes, racking my brains to recollect what I'd read, I felt as though I'd been listening to a conversation in a far-off room. One I thought I'd been in on, only to discover that all I could hear were its most distant squeaks and shuffles. Then, nearly a year and a half after Jesse's birth, I realized I could again turn things I had read over in my mind. Not always yet, but sometimes. I was back in on the conversation.

So I was on the lookout for allies. People who'd behaved as I had, or been treated as I had, and found a tale to tell about it. I needed to make imaginary liaisons. Those I found are all a far cry from my own, but, still and all, enough. Margery Kempe was one of the first. She found divine method in her fourteenth-century madness. It seems astonishing that the first autobiography ever written in the English language should begin with a terrifying account of postpartum psychosis. Margery Kempe saw devils and described herself in a state of deluded sin. But her description sounded all too familiar to me, of someone in terrible despair, in a place where nobody and nothing could impinge on her appalling isolation.

The spirits who called her to action at the beginning of her autobiography seem close kin to those that whispered to me at the start of mine. They made her bite "her own hand so violently that the mark could be seen for the rest of her life," just like the marks on mine. They made her tear "the skin on her body near her heart with her nails," just as I did mine. Like me she was prevented from doing something worse. In her case, the only thing they could do was tie her up, both day and night.

Better the devil you know than the devil you don't, so, like me, Kempe made her madness central to her life's project. It became a step on her way to holiness. When I read *The Book of Mary Kempe,* I felt oddly outraged by the way she makes this terrifying breakdown into just a scrap of trauma, the first, tiny part of her pilgrimage into mysticism. It occupies only the first three out of three hundred pages. My breakdown held the story of my life, though I didn't yet know how, and I felt it should do the same for everyone else, even for this mystic from six hundred years ago.

Nevertheless, Margery Kempe stands in my imaginary company as a kind of founding mother. Somebody who found a way to own their state of mind, and in their own words.

When my mother pointed out to me that the woman in *The Yellow Wallpaper* had just had a baby, I reread it. It's the story of a woman going mad in a room by herself and gradually inhabiting and becoming inhabited by its lurid wallpaper. My mother had been reading it as an undergraduate student shortly after Jesse was born, just as I had ten years before. Then I had had no children and my life was organized around quite different concerns. Reading it this second time was a different event.

I was struck immediately by how much is done to infantilize the woman in the story. It is she, not her baby, who is put in the nursery and patronized by her arrogantly concerned doctor husband. He treats her as a small child and refuses to listen to her seriously. And in the course of the story she becomes absorbed into her hallucinations, of a woman both entrapped by and escaping from the insidious, grotesquely fecund wallpaper. Gradually she tears it from the walls until finally her husband finds her creeping around the room, locked into delusions that now offer her a truer version of her life than he can.

During my first hour in the psychiatric hospital, the thing that shocked me most was the paper on the walls of the bedroom I was to inhabit. As far as I can recall, it had a brown floral pattern. Above one bed it had been torn, from above our heads down to waist level. The nurse didn't tell me that day that it had been torn by the woman I was to be sharing the room with. It was like a sign written on the walls, that here I was inhabiting a place very different from any I had known. And I didn't yet know how far I was inside it or outside. The tears and scratches on the walls were marks of violent protest — defacing the scant attempt to give a homely aura to this hospital room. Nothing was sacred, not even the bland, institutional décor of the ward. A woman might attack anything in this second confinement, giving birth this time to her own madness. I was horrified by the idea that I, too, might be capable of that kind of behavior.

In *The Yellow Wallpaper* the woman's voice of calm explanation is terrifyingly at odds with the rising pitch of madness. I never suffered delusions like hers, but I remember well my sense that my actions — the head-banging, the mutilation of my arms and hands, the attempts to scorch myself — were the logical response to my predicament, though I couldn't explain the logic to anyone else. Charlotte Perkins Gilman's story manages that impossible divide very well. And though we know her protagonist is seeing things, what she sees is a kind of insight into her situation as a woman condescended to but not listened to.

Gilman's story suddenly took a new shape for me when I read it this second time. The doctor husband's wish to suppress his wife's "imaginative power and habit of storymaking" for fear of the "excited fancies" it will lead her into reminds me of one well-intentioned piece of advice that came my way in the hospital. One of the nurses told me: "Stop trying to work it all out; it will get you nowhere." Yet nowhere was where I already was.

Reading her story again after my own breakdown, I wanted to know more about Gilman, and read Jeffrey

Berman's *The Talking Cure*. Having learned a little of what she experienced, I was taken aback by how strongly I could identify with her. After her daughter was born, Gilman, like me, found she could neither read nor write, nor get out of bed. Increasingly all she did was cry. She couldn't make herself happy and she blamed herself for her misery. Eventually she took the psychiatrist S. Weir Mitchell's once famous and now notorious rest-cure. After a month in his sanatorium she returned home with the injunction to live "as domestic a life as possible. Have your child with you all the time . . . Lie down an hour after each meal. Have but two hours' intellectual life a day. And never touch pen, brush, or pencil as long as you live."

After trying to follow Mitchell's directions for three months, Gilman said she "went nearly mad." The shape of her near-madness and the shape of mine, also after leaving the hospital, seem very alike. Gilman made herself a rag doll, hung it from a doorknob, and would play with it at length, though if she had to dress her own child it left her "shaking and crying." I, too, was frightened of being left alone in the house with my children. Not because of what I might do to them, or they to me, but because then I could not escape from the knowledge that this was my life now, and there was no getting away from it. Gilman "would crawl into remote closets and under beds — to hide from the grinding pressure of that profound distress." I would do the same. I can still chart my own house by the corners and small spaces in each room that I could hunch myself into. Gilman would sit blankly, turning her head one way and then the other, unable to escape her mental agony. For over a year and a half I banged my head against different walls, usually structural ones because they are harder in our house, searching for some relief from the rage inside it. Gilman's terrible torpor lifted only when she ignored the advice of her psychiatrist and began, once again, to write. Like Gilman, I can command my life in words, where I was lost to myself before I found them.

❖   ❖   ❖

Sometimes when I go to write, I encourage myself with a small sentence of exhortation. This often takes the shape of a quiet muttering beneath my breath as I drag my feet up the stairs to my study against the inertia that is always lurking beneath the staircase. It's odd how unwilling I am to do one of the things that gives me the greatest pleasure. To visit that place where I discover my thoughts. Maybe, though, this old familiar comes from the same place as the leaching blankness that seemed to sap all the words when both my body and my mind were flattened by blank despair. Then inertia seemed to drain even the colors from the air around me and I could no more describe how I felt than fly. When I read William Styron's *Darkness Visible,* my first feeling was relief, that someone else, a writer no less, found his state of mind nearly impossible to articulate.

Adam gave me Styron's book during one of my rare unaccompanied visits to London. I'd started writing my own story by now and began to read his with that familiar suppressed panic, that he might have got there before me and used up all the words. I read it on the subway, heading north from central London at the same time as a crowd of soccer fans on their way to Wembley. Styron's interior dialogue seemed more alarming than all the striped-scarf ranters. Their shouts faded to nothing beside the pain he tries to describe. He compares it to drowning and suffocation, but says these images are off the mark. I understood his predicament. The comparisons I found for my own despair, like Styron's, so often veered off into terrible ultimatums. What I felt like seemed beyond living with, yet here I was, alive. Styron had never drowned or suffocated, but he could find no other way of wording it. I finished the book before reaching my destination.

I was very thin during that subway ride and I wore my hat low over my brow to cover a wound on my forehead that I'd made with a stone. Nineteen months after Jesse's birth and I could allow no food into me until evening fell. I'd bought some jeans that day and, standing in front of the mirror in the shop, I wondered whether the slender reflection before me was something I loved or hated. But whatever it was that stopped me from eating and made me gash my skin open, I knew it had to do with who or what I felt myself to be. It did not depend, as I read that day in Styron's little book, on how my synapses were functioning.

It was a relief to come across somebody who was used to getting his way with words, not being able to find them. But I was dismayed by the explanation Styron comes up with for it all. For most of his book he insists that depression is all in the body. It's a disease, an illness, a disorder, a question of neurotransmitters and hormones, something you leave to the biochemist rather than the biographer or autobiographer. No one, neither him nor anyone else, he says, will ever learn about their depression, since "madness results from an aberrant biochemical process." Styron becomes a sophist with remarks like these, describing modern psychiatry as a conveniently unprovable science, on which nevertheless he can hang an explanation of his own predicament.

Only at the very end does he hint at a different story, the kind I needed and found. There he concedes, unwillingly, that perhaps his suicidal depression arose out of a terrible sense of loss. Possibly if Styron had allowed himself to, if he'd given himself a little more space, he might have understood his breakdown not so much as a clinical condition but as the shape he found for his life's grief. But maybe that's also why he keeps his book so short. It leaves him no time to look at his shape in the mirror.

That same March I sat at my kitchen table one bleary afternoon and started to read another book shown me by another friend. Bridget this time. A handful of pages later the story had me in its thrall. My children swirled around my legs with their toys, demanding my scrutiny every few minutes. They knew, as they always do so fast, that I was somehow abstracted. And, not content with the froth and skim of my attention, they made my reading that afternoon impossible.

During the next week I consumed this book with a terrific hunger. I read Marie Cardinal's *The Words to Say It* in the same way that I had read about the lives of the virtuous years before. The symptoms of her distress acted on my mind just as miracles had in the past. Having only recently begun my own psychotherapy, I found her conversion to psychoanalysis compelling. Her writing had me hooked. I had begun my own talking and writing cure when I read this book. I was already in search of my own words. What Cardinal's account confirmed for me, beyond anything else, was the license to be interested in the invention that is your own life. She'd done it, so could I.

In her first analytic session, Cardinal's analyst says he's not interested in the physical symptom that, for her, legitimizes her own madness. For a moment, the briefest psychoanalytic second, she is shocked, as though he had struck her across the face. But his rebuff liberates her attention — she is free for the first time to ignore her body and the mysterious bleeding, like a continuous period, that has afflicted her for so long. And it tells her that there is something more important, and therefore better defended and harder to reach, that he is interested in.

Cardinal recounts her profound ambivalence in giving up the security of her illness. To do so she has to allow the history behind it to surface. She describes both the sour and the sweet taste of her childhood as her analysis progresses, and most particularly the figure her mother cut in her heart from earliest memory. Her analysis veers, from season to season, between dreamlike conjurings, high-pressure diving into memory, murderous fury, exhilaration, lassitude, blankness, bewilderment, pleasure, and lucidity. Out of all this she finds words to say it. She discovers she can write and does so.

I have found it liberating not to be ill. But it has taken me a long time to give up the bitter smell of my own misery. Sometimes still, it seems most inviting. Cardinal's book was an inspiration, like somebody whispering to me that that bitterness and gall might be the very place to start writing, and who knew what might rise out of the paper.

Cardinal describes her own censorship of her past. Slowly, through her analysis, she survives her own memories, then reappropriates them. Somebody told me recently that Cardinal now says that much of what she has put into *The Words to Say It* is made up. For a moment I was dismayed. But then I realized that it doesn't really matter. What did matter was that when I started to trust my own words, both in my therapy and in my writing, I read a book in which someone else told how they learned to find and to lean on theirs.

When I was admitted to the psychiatric hospital, in the course of taking down my "history," several psychiatrists asked me what I had been writing my thesis about. Some, it would seem, listened to my answers more carefully than others. When my notes were sent to me, there was a letter attached at the back that had been sent by Dr. A.'s senior houseman to my GP in mid-January, a month after I had been discharged. In the course of my "personal history," I am described as returning to the university "to do a PhD in American Post-Elizabethan Bishops, which has recently been submitted." I was amused by this misreading of my medical notes, but also dismayed. I now know that the substance of what I said didn't matter while I was in the hospital. But it is still galling to find my intellectual lifework for the previous five years described as a piece of remote ecclesiastical history.

On my first meeting with Dr. A., she asked me what I had been writing my thesis about. She listened a little harder than her houseman had done, but only to tell me of her distaste for another writer. When I said it was about a modern American woman poet, she asked me which one. I told her and she thanked God it wasn't that Sylvia Plath again. She'd had enough, she said, of her student patients coming in obsessed with Sylvia Plath. Hugh remembers this exchange, not me. But having re-read *The Bell Jar* recently, I think Dr. A.'s dislike of Plath was well founded. Had they met, their feelings might have been more eye-for-an-eye than eye-to-eye.

The first time I read *The Bell Jar* was as a second-year undergraduate. I studied it in the same American literature course as I had *The Yellow Wallpaper*. The course was taught by Hermione, someone I had not yet met, but who was to become one of my closest friends. When I returned to Plath's novel ten years later, I knew I was the same person I'd been then. But how differently that twenty-one-year-old would have described herself from the person aged thirty-one. Then Plath's novel seemed a kind of beautifully crafted, traumatic artifact, not like an experience I'd ever have myself. Now I've lived under my own bell jar and the metaphor no longer seems overdone.

I had to return to *The Bell Jar*, not because I particularly identify with Plath's heroine Esther or with Plath herself, but because Plath, or her book (it's hard to know which or both), has become such an archetype, such a loaded figure. How could any English-speaking woman writer consider mental illness, mental hospitals, ECT, the language of despair, without at least curtseying briefly to Sylvia Plath? Here I was, a greenhorn, working on her first book. Maybe I could appropriate this dead American poet as a symbolic figure for my own narrative. In fact, when I tried writing about *The*

Bell Jar, what came out was a "mine's bigger than hers" comparison mixed with a bit of literary criticism. So I noted that Esther gets less ECT than me, but hers is nastier. That I have more drugs than her and that she gets psychotherapy without asking. And I describe Esther's, or do I mean Plath's, determination to hold on to her nightmare experience as something I, too, know about.

It's funny how fiercely the early readers of my book have wanted me to keep, or get rid of, my reading of *The Bell Jar.* I haven't quite done either. Because although I slip the novel somewhat self-consciously in among the books I've needed near, re-reading it marked an important step for me. It was like an announcement to myself that I, too, would craft my distress into something others could hold.

I've found it difficult, writing about the language in which other people compose their drastic discomposure. But it has been important to me to read these stories, maybe for the same reason that I used to read about the lives of terrifying and godly Christians. Then I sought the example of men and women as a spur to good works. When I started writing, it was a spur to good words I was looking for. The books I've described form an oddly complete composite shape in my mind now. They are the ones I came across when I needed to, those in which I found the encouragement to give voice. I find I use my own memories like a series of echograms, trying to establish the contours of somebody else's plunge and rise. Though I might have nothing in common with them but this, it's been part of my journey back to want to hear tales from other continents, other voyages to the underworld.

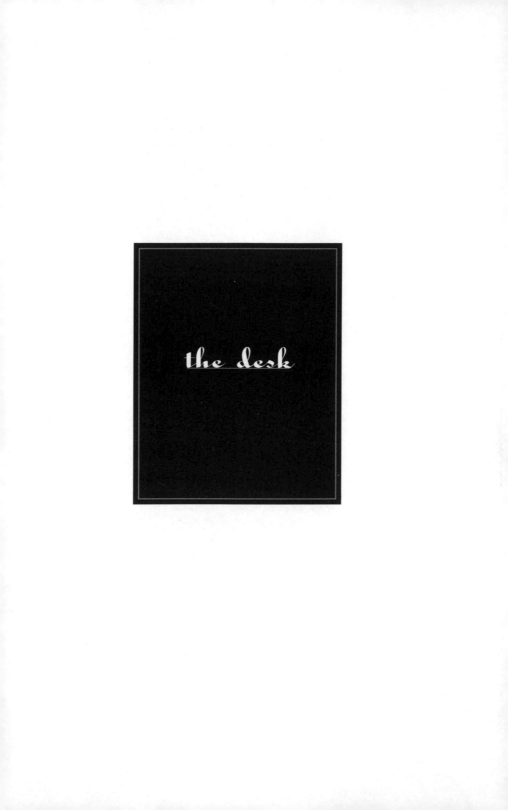

the desk

LITTLE HAS CHANGED on my desk
since Eliza's birth, or so it might seem. Covered with books,
papers, notes to myself, and "littered with old correspon-
dences" (Elizabeth Bishop's phrase), it looks much the same
as ever. I sit facing a wall that plays host to a rising staircase
of different women. The angel Gabriel telling Mary the un-
believable is repeated maybe twenty times on postcards from
low on the flank of wall to the left of my desk. This heap of
annunciations is interrupted only by a photograph stuck
between Piero della Francesca and Jan van Eyck, of me minutes after Eliza's birth. I am red-faced and euphoric, bloody-
armed as though I had massacred, not given birth to, an

innocent. But cradled against my balloon of a breast is a tiny, white-fisted figure. Her hair is still plastered to her head and she has blood on her forehead. With her eyes tight shut she looks as though she is making a wish.

Then, with her head still ducked low, the Virgin Mary, absorbed in quiet apprehension, gives way to Eleonora Duse, Greta Garbo, Simone de Beauvoir, Virginia Woolf, Salome, Martina Navratilova, Emmeline Pankhurst, Anna Akhmatova, the other Fiona Shaw, and a host of other women who bear silent witness to my efforts. They seem to encounter camera, paintbrush, or sculptor's chisel with quite different dreams of a future. Some dance, others are seated, some cradle children. Each, to my eye, is handsome. Each, most importantly, seems in possession of herself.

As the stair of pictures descends above my head, these women, these alter egos who make such figures of my fantasies, give way to incidental images of my own life. There is a photograph of me aged three in a red mackintosh and Wellington boots. My mother leans out of a car window, smiling in the late 1950s at my father seated on its bonnet. Eliza, perhaps two months old, sleeps on her sleeping father's chest. My sister Jules is caught against her will shortly before one of her extended flights to elsewhere, her hair cropped short in anticipation of the Indonesian sun. I am reading Alice Munro's *Lives of Girls and Women* with Eliza, a few months old, asleep on my lap, sated with milk.

There is a photograph, a little out of focus, of one of my favorite birds, a tern, dropping, wings tucked, into the sea off Brighton pier. My mother smiles to me, with the shadow of an Italian medieval arch caught by the February sun on the wall behind her. In a composite of two photographs I and my friend Adam sit at each end of a table in Ireland, the teapot and tablecloth caught at an angle in the join between pictures. We have been captured in mock frivolity during serious conversation about my draft thesis, a pile of papers in front of us both. Hugh figures everywhere.

One of the last photographs to find its place on this wall shows me with Eliza and Jesse, squatting in front of a dark shadow of a tree trunk. The canopy of leaves from this vast tree is a blur behind and just visible low on the trunk is the dark, slender outline of a half-grown cat. As a child I used to climb high into this copper beech tree, sometimes with a book, until I was invisible to the world. It was the shape beyond my bedroom window throughout my childhood, and it marked out for me something that never changed, though its branches were sculpted by the seasons. My face is mournful in the picture. The house was sold last summer when the photograph was taken, and with it my capacity to call the tree my own. The picture bears witness to my grief at parting.

Jesse didn't feature as a small baby above my desk until recently because I couldn't bear the pain that that still tiny face reminded me of. But then she noticed her own absence and requested that I make her present. So the most recent photograph is of Jesse in my arms when she was perhaps three months old. Something has caught her eye and she gazes out of the photograph. My eyes look down, out of the camera's lens, to my daughter. I know, because Hugh has told me, that I couldn't bear to face the camera then. My face seems calm, bleached. There is little to betray me. But

the inscrutability of the photograph makes me queasy, as
though I have been caught out in a lie.

Then there are my stones. When I was a child I used to
collect the small brown and yellow shells I found on the
beaches in Devon. I would glaze them and put them in glass
jars. My passion was in the getting of them. Once collected
they lost their potency and I ignored them. Now I have
stones, also garnered from the tide. There is a bowl of small,
black, smooth ones on my desk that I found on a beach in
Ireland last summer. Their contours are impeccably approx-
imate, drawing close to diamonds, squares, triangles, and
ovals. Each is distinguished, perhaps by a fleck of abrasion on
its surface, or by a slight failure of geometric resolve, the
third side of a triangle folding into two, or a rectangle with
a corner missing. I make pictures on top of my desk with
these stones, forming them into composite designs, or faces.
I have added to them one piece of square slate, in danger of
sharding itself, from the beach in Devon where my accumulating began.

The other stones about my desk are much larger, carrying a dubious alibi as paperweights. These, too, I have gathered from a beach in the west of Ireland. When I hold one,
it brings to mind a place where I can hear myself think.
There is always the roar of the water breaking on the steeply
pitched shingle, and it is easy to be lost to the sound of other
people's voices but to find one's own. So, mindful of that
other place, I use these stony echoes to anchor my thoughts
in a small village in the north of England.

I have a snake, too, on my desk now. It is an Indian
cobra's head in old bronze, perhaps two inches high. I often

stroke the curve of its hood, perhaps to coax honey from the gall of memories, as I managed to coax love for snakes out of fear when I was small. Also a small branch from the beech tree that was mine. There is a photograph of my father I remember being taken when I was about seven, a box of pens and pencils, hand cream, a dictionary, my laptop technology, and a line of books.

Before I acquired my first computer I used to write my essays with a pen, only typing up the completed version. My handwritten script always appeared like a kind of chaos, with paragraphs scored out, added in the margin, apparently jumbled and confused, with asterisks all around like dubious stars. And I had to trust that I had created something coherent in my convoluted, inconsistent hand. Until I had typed it up, I never knew quite what shape it had taken. Witnessing my writing technique one day, while I was studying for an M.A. in Brighton, Hugh wrote a limerick. It is still stuck on the wall above my desk, to the right of Salome with head in hand, and beneath Caravaggio's exquisite red-haired Maddalena:

> *There was a young girl with an essay*
> *whose writing was dauntingly messy.*
> *When they said "What's your game?"*
> *She said "Finn's the name*
> *and this will soon be a most finnished essay."*

My writing technique hasn't changed. When I complete a piece of writing, I still don't know how it will all add up until I read it at the end. I can't hold the different parts in mind at the same time, or assemble them mentally into a particular shape. Now, as I describe all I see about my desk, I am aware that many of the preoccupations I hold most dear are figured here. But before I began to assemble them in these paragraphs, I had no idea of this. My desk seems to have become a brilliantly tangible metaphor for my mind, the kind of accumulation that I need to have around me in this place that I call my very own.

I've talked very little about my children. My study is the place I go to to leave them behind and, curiously, I seem to have done this in my writing too. A while ago Eliza was playing a let's-pretend game in which she took all the parts. When she started pretending to be me, she hid under a blanket and imitated me typing on my keyboard. I've written much of this book in the afternoon while the children watch *Sesame Street* on television, recorded from earlier in the day. This afternoon hour is one I can snatch possibly three times during the week. After setting them up with apples and rice cakes in front of the television, without stopping to do anything else, I climb the stairs to my study and face my own music.

When *Sesame Street* is over, they come to find me. First Jesse, then Eliza, veer into the room without checking their pace and my time is up. Sometime I can snatch a few more minutes while they play with a basket of pebbles and old marbles on the windowsill. But once that game is over, it's their turn at the keyboard. Eliza likes to tap in some names, Eliza, Jesse, Daddy or Hugh, Mummy or Finn, Pangur (our cat), and sundry others. Then they each tell a story, always of children and often of dragons and princesses, which I type for them. The story is anything from three lines long, and when it has ended, nothing I can do will persuade either to extend it. It is finished. This is one Eliza wrote when she was nearly four, just as I was writing this ending:

> *Once upon a time a tiny girl called Mummy when she was five or six or seven and she lived in a house with Eliza and Jesse and Daddy. She had her birthday cake and she had a big party. And then the only thing she could do was walk and talk and eat and go asleep. And then people knew that. She was in Africa and the story was written in African and that's why you can't understand it. I'm bored of telling stories. That's the end of the story.*

When I've printed their stories out, they run down the stairs, sheet in hand, proud of what they have made, keen to show it to Hugh when he returns in the evening. I know how they feel.

Other than these snatched times, I have four and a half hours of potential writing time during the week, when the children are looked after elsewhere. And I have a morning during the weekend whenever it is possible. For the rest, I am a mother, exhausted and exhilarated by turns. My children can drive me into distracted fury faster than I would have thought possible. Jesse's refusal to eat another spoonful of cereal can leave me close to tears. Eliza wheeling her trike around the kitchen table in February, singing "Away in a Manger" very loudly again and again, in spite of my embargo on carols after January and my crescendo of requests for her to stop, makes me wish in a shrill voice that Herod had had his way. Then, of course, her curiosity makes me wish I had never mentioned infanticide.

It is tiring to have to negotiate each move of each day. I have to coax my kids into coats, persuade them to sit on chairs during meals, bribe Eliza to go for a walk, though she never stops running at home, lure Jesse to bed even when she's sleeping standing up, and so on. And I find a lot of this very boring. As I listen to myself I loathe the monotony of what I seem to have to say.

My children seem to possess me body and soul much of the time. But part of this possession consists of their capacity to move me utterly and to make me laugh. Their excitement with the world I've borne them into is infectious. They make me see things differently and their boundless curiosity keeps me stretched to the limit of my imagination. They don't suffer yet from that grown-up propriety which decrees that some things are not interesting. And I am still taken aback by the love they command. As my rage rises faster at Eliza and Jesse than at anyone else, just so it drops. I cannot sustain it for long and usually find my remorse is way in advance of theirs.

❖　　❖　　❖

When I began writing this book, I did so in the effort to shore myself up against the whirling chaos of my mind. I was in fear of disintegration, though I couldn't, and still can't, describe what I mean by that. I had no idea that my terror would give birth to a book. What has been important has been the act of turning blankness and confusion into narrative coherence, however provisional. And though I started by doing that with my experience after Jesse's birth, I quickly found myself doing the same thing with my earlier life. Though it's not effaced from my memory in quite the same way as the more recent past, I had no sense of coherence for any of it. I didn't know, before I began, how to go about making it out.

When I read what I wrote last year, I am relieved that I have nearly finished this writing. I don't think I could bear to do that work of remembering again. Were I to try to write about my life again in a few years' time, it would come out very differently. If I think of my past as a kind of glossary that I hold in my head, then I know that the words and memories I uncover as glosses on the present will change month by month and year by year. Now that I'm ending the book, I'm trying to ask myself where it has brought me to. I am still at my desk, just where I started, but I think I have also traveled a considerable distance. One of those journeys in the mind that Jesse and Eliza are so keen on.

I can't offer conclusions, because, patently, nothing is finished. Looking back over my writing, I can see it as a process, in which I am trying to find a way of telling something that expands beyond the page even as I write it. I've read my medical and nursing notes, experiencing my own life in the third person. I've pondered the languages other people write in to describe, as Marie Cardinal did, what it is like to break down and then find their own words to say it. I've talked with many other women who, like me, found themselves traumatized after the birth of a baby. I've grappled with psychiatry, trying to recognize my own predicament in its language while maintaining my distance from its coercive jargon. And I have read any books or articles I have come across about "postpartum depression," listening for a common tune. My effort to find a language for my own experience is charted through each of these negotiations. In the end, nobody can voice my life to me except myself.

Sometimes still I feel all too close to the person curled up in the corner after Jesse's birth. But that intimacy no longer strangles me. Sometimes I can stroke the snake, not only let it mesmerize me with fear. I don't beat myself up as often. I don't throw up as often, though I am still too thin. I'm no longer terrified of being in my own home. I want my life now, and the people in it. And I know I want to go on writing. A detective novel next, perhaps, replete with conclusions.

I seem a different person to the one encountered two and a half years ago. So I am told. Not, you understand, that I am not myself. That I remain. And certainly I have recovered something vital. I like to laugh again, play with my children, watch and live in the world beyond my own mind. I take pleasure. But whatever was laid bare after Jesse's birth is still close beneath my skin, and somehow I need it to be, though it may not be so visible to others. When I am unhappy I often seem to myself like a mourner without an object for my grief. Until I discover and understand that object, I will go on keening, in the privacy of my own person. I'm not ready nor able, yet, to give up possession of my own desperation.

But I don't descend into it as I used to — not as often and not for such long stretches. Nothing like, yet all too like. All these changes seem terribly conditional, frail — except of course for my book. That is out of me. I've said now what I didn't know was there to be said before. It sits in front of me on my desk, so much confusion and mess neatly piled and printed.

BIBLIOGRAPHY

Berman, Jeffrey. *The Talking Cure: Literary Representations of Psychoanalysis*. New York: New York University Press, 1985.

Bishop, Elizabeth. *The Complete Poems 1927–1979*. New York: Farrar, Straus & Giroux, 1984.

Bloom, Amy. *Come to Me*. New York: HarperCollins, 1994.

Brockington, I. F. and R. Kumar, *Motherhood and Mental Illness*. San Antonio, Texas: Psychological Corp., 1982.

Cardinal, Marie. *The Words to Say It*. Cambridge, Ma.: Van Vector & Goodheart, 1983.

Clare, Anthony. *Psychiatry in Dissent*. London: Tavistock, 1976; rpt. Routledge, 1992.

Cobb, John. *Babyshock: A Mother's First Five Years*. London: Hutchinson, 1980.

Comport, Maggie. *Surviving Motherhood: Coping with Postnatal Depression.* Bath, England: Ashgrove Press, 1990.

Cooper, David. *Psychiatry and Anti-Psychiatry.* London: Tavistock, 1967.

Cox, J. L. *Postnatal Depression: A Guide for Health Professionals.* Edinburgh: Churchill Livingstone, 1986.

Cozens, Jenny. *Nervous Breakdown.* London: Piatkus, 1988; rpt. 1993.

Dalton, Katharina. *Depression After Childbirth.* Oxford: Oxford University Press, 1980; 3rd edition, 1996.

Dana, Mira, and Marilyn Lawrence. *Women's Secret Disorder: A New Understanding of Bulimia.* London: Grafton, 1988; rpt. 1989.

Dickinson, Julie. "Sharing the Pain of Motherhood," *Nursing Times* 86 No. 39 (1990): 36–38.

Dix, Carol. *The New Mother Syndrome: Coping with Post-natal Stress and Depression.* New York: Pocket, 1988.

Frame, Janet. *Faces in the Water.* New York: Braziller, 1982.

———. *Janet Frame: An Autobiography,* 3 vols. New York: Braziller, 1991.

Freud, Sigmund. *On Metapsychology.* Harmondsworth, England: Penguin, 1984.

Gelder, M., D. Gath, and R. Mayou. *Concise Oxford Textbook of Psychiatry.* Oxford: Oxford University Press, 1994.

Gilman, Charlotte Perkins. *The Yellow Wallpaper.* New York: Feminist Press, 1988.

Gorey, Edward. *The Listing Attic and The Unstrung Harp; or, Mr Earbrass Writes a Novel.* London: Abelard–Schuman, 1974.

Holden, Jenifer. "She Just Listened." *Community Outlook.*
July 1987.

Holmes Coleman, Emily. *The Shutter of Snow.* New York:
Dalkey Archive Press, 1997.

Hughes, Jennifer. *An Outline of Modern Psychiatry.*
Chichester, England: Wiley, 1991.

Kaysen, Susanna. *Girl, Interrupted.* New York: Vintage, 1994.

Kempe, Margery. *The Book of Margery Kempe: The
Autobiography of the Madwoman of God.* Liguori, Mo.:
Triumph Books, 1995.

Kendell, R. E. et al. "Mood Changes in the First Three
Weeks After Childbirth." *Journal of Affective Disorders* 3
(1981): 317–26.

Klein, Melanie. *Selected Melanie Klein.* edited by Juliet
Mitchell. New York: Free Press, 1987.

Kumar, R. "Childbirth and Mental Illness." *Triangle* 29 No.
2/3 (1990): 73–81.

Kumar, R., and I. F. Brockington. *Motherhood and Mental
Illness 2: Causes and Consequences.* London: John Wright,
1988.

Laing, R. D. *The Divided Self.* New York: Viking, 1991.

Laing, R. D., and A. Esterson. *Sanity, Madness and the
Family.* New York: Basic, 1971.

Marks, Jenny. "Maternal Depression: Who Is at Risk?"
Health Visitor 53 (January 1980): 7–9.

Marshall, Fiona. *Coping with Postnatal Depression: Why It
Happens and How to Overcome It.* London: Sheldon, 1993.

McCabe, Patrick. *Carn.* New York: Bantam, 1997.

Millett, Kate. *The Loony-Bin Trip.* New York: Simon &
Schuster, 1990.

Nickson, Elizabeth. *The Monkey-Puzzle Tree.* London: Bloomsbury, 1995.

Oakley, Ann. *Women Confined: Towards a Sociology of Childbirth.* New York: Schocken, 1980.

Parker, Rozsika. *Torn in Two: The Experience of Maternal Ambivalence.* London: Virago, 1995.

Plath, Sylvia. *The Bell Jar.* New York: HarperCollins, 1996.

——. *Journals of Sylvia Plath.* New York: Ballantine, 1991.

Porter, Roy. *A Social History of Madness: Stories of the Insane.* London: Weidenfeld & Nicolson, 1989.

Pound, A. et al. "The Impact of Maternal Depression on Young Children." *Recent Results in Developmental Psychopathology, Journal of Child Psychology and Psychiatry* (1985, supp. 4): 3–10.

Price, Jane. *Motherhood: What It Does to Your Mind.* London: Pandora, 1988.

Rich, Adrienne. *Of Woman Born: Motherhood as Experience and Institution.* New York: Norton, 1976.

Rogers, Jane. *The Ice Is Singing.* London: Faber, 1987.

Sapsted, Anne-Marie. *Banish Post-Baby Blues.* Wellingborough, England: Thorsons, 1990.

Sedgwick, Peter. *Psycho Politics.* London: Pluto Press, 1982.

Showalter, Elaine. *The Female Malady: Women, Madness and English Culture, 1830–1980.* New York: Pantheon, 1986.

Snaith, R. P. "Pregnancy-Related Psychiatric Disorder." *British Journal of Hospital Medicine* 29 no. 5 (1983): 450–56.

Stevens, Wallace. *Collected Poems.* New York: Vintage, 1990.

Styron, William. *Darkness Visible.* New York: Random House, 1990.

Weekes, Claire. *Self-Help for Your Nerves.* Oxford: Isis, 1986.

Welburn, Vivienne. *Postnatal Depression.* Manchester, England: Manchester University Press, 1980.

White, Antonia. *Beyond the Glass.* London: Virago, 1979, rpt. 1991.

ACKNOWLEDGMENTS

I am grateful for the support, encouragement, friendship, suggestions, cautions, and conversation of many different people, and especially for the generosity of those people whose words I have quoted. I would especially like to thank the following:

Clare Alexander, Chris Botham, Chris Defty, Judy Donovan, Michael Fend, Ann Finch, Tim Gates, Anthea Gomez, Frances Gordon, Kate Griffin, Victoria Hobbs, Sue Hogge, Lou Hoole, Gilli Jackson, Lawrence Jacobsen, Amanda Lillie, Paul Munden, Michael Neve, Anthony O'Carroll, Jan Pitkin, Felicity Riddy, Nicole Ward-Jouve, Debbie Waxenberg, Heather Williams, and Helen Wilmerding.

Claire Delpech, Channi Kumar, and Merton Sandler have been generous with their time and expertise. Ruthie

Petrie gave me the encouragement I needed to go on with the book at a time when I though it might never see the light of publication.

I am grateful for the support of my friends Bridget Bennett, Sue Fothergill, Sara Perrin, and Michelle Willett, who gave me their humor and affection when all around I was losing mine. And to Jacqueline Rose and Kate Weaver, who have been unstinting in their support for my high and low selves.

I am particularly indebted to Hermione Lee and Adam Phillips, my first readers, for their sustained, affectionate, and intellectual encouragement. Without their provocation I might never have forced my own hand. To my agent, Alexandra Pringle, I owe a debt I could never have envisaged when I first climbed the multiple flights to her office. To my editor, Michael Moore, my thanks for his conviction that this book was worth publishing on the other side of the Atlantic, and for his care in doing so.

My family — Sarah, John, Jules, and Lucy Edington and Mike Shaw — have shown love and relative forbearance in the face of it all, far beyond the call of duty. And without my precious daughters, Eliza and Jesse, this book would have been something else and I thank them for their vigorous pleasures and child insights that have brought me up short when I thought I knew enough.

Last of all, to Hugh Haughton, who, from my first sentence, discussed it all, agreed, agreed to differ, and joked with me, I owe more than can be said without embarrassment.

A NOTE ON THE AUTHOR

Fiona Shaw grew up in London and lives in the
north of England where she is now working on
her first novel.

❖

A NOTE ON THE BOOK

This book was composed by Steerforth Press
using a digital version of Bembo, a typeface
produced by Monotype in 1929 and based on
.he designs of Francesco Griffo, Venice 1499.
The book was printed on acid free papers and
bound by Quebecor Printing ~ Book Press
Inc. of North Brattleboro, Vermont.